D0065270

Evidence-Based Behavioral Health Practices for Older Adults

About the Editors

Sue E. Levkoff, ScD, is an associate professor in psychiatry at Brigham and Women's Hospital and an associate professor in the Department of Social Medicine, Harvard Medical School. She currently serves as the director for the Positive Aging Resource Center, a national technical assistance center for enhancing behavioral health services for older adults. Dr. Levkoff also directs the Coordinating Center for a national study that evaluates effectiveness of the innovative geriatric mental health service programs in primary care clinics across the country. She was former president of the Association of Geriatric Education Centers, and is currently director of the Harvard Partners Geriatric Education Center.

Hongtu Chen, PhD, is a senior research scientist at Brigham and Women's Hospital and an instructor in the Department of Psychiatry, Harvard Medical School. He currently serves as an implementation specialist at the Positive Aging Resource Center. He is a psychologist trained in mental health and health service research. Dr. Chen has extensive experience with developing, implementing, and evaluating mental health services for aging populations in general, and ethnic Asian American older adults in particular. His research interests and publications focus on geriatric mental health, culture-bound syndromes of depression, service planning and evaluation, and implementation of evidence-based practices in mental health care.

Jane E. Fisher, PhD, is a professor of clinical psychology and former director of clinical training at the University of Nevada, Reno. She is Executive Director of the Nevada Caregiver Support Center, a statewide program funded by the Nevada Division for Aging Services that provides training in evidence-based behavioral health care practices for elderly persons and caregiving families. Dr. Fisher is a technical advisor on evidence-based practice for the Positive Aging Resource Center. Dr. Fisher's research interests include behavioral health and aging, applied behavior analysis, and the integration of evidence-based behavioral health care in primary and long-term care settings. Her research on the development of restraint-free interventions for elderly persons with cognitive disorders is funded by the National Institute on Aging.

John S. McIntyre, MD, is the vice president for Behavioral Health and chair of the Department of Psychiatry and Behavioral Health at Unity Health System in Rochester, New York, and clinical professor of psychiatry at the University of Rochester. He has served on the National Alliance of the Mentally Ill National Advisory Council Stigma Campaign. He was former president of American Psychiatric Association (APA). He currently is the senior delegate from the APA to the American Medical Association and chair of the APA Steering Committee on Practice Guidelines. His clinical and research interests include the development and use of practice guidelines, integration of psychiatry and primary care, and the involvement of patients and patient advocates in the planning and evaluation of clinical services.

Evidence-Based Behavioral Health Practices for Older Adults

A *Guide to* Implementation

Edited by

Sue E. Levkoff, ScD
Hongtu Chen, PhD
Jane E. Fisher, PhD
John S. McIntyre, MD

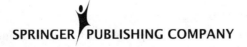

SPRINGER PUBLISHING COMPANY

New York

Springer Publishing Company, Inc.
11 West 42nd Street
New York, NY 10036

Acquisitions Editor: Helvi Gold
Production Editor: Gail F. Farrar
Cover design: Mimi Flow
Composition: Publishers' Design and Production Services, Inc.

06 07 08 09 10 / 5 4 3 2 1

Library of Congress Cataloging-in-Publication Data

Evidence-based behavioral health practices for older adults : a guide to implementation / edited by Sue Levkoff . . . [et al.].
    p. cm.
    Includes bibliographical references and index.
    ISBN 0-8261-6965-1
    1. Older people—mental health. 2. Older people—mental health services. 3. Preventive mental health services for older people. 4. Evidence-based psychiatry. I. Levkoff, Sue.

RA564.8.E95 2006
618.97'689—dc22

                                                    2006044256

Contents

Contributors ix

Foreword xi
Patrick J. Kennedy

Acknowledgments xiii

Introduction xv
Sue E. Levkoff, Hongtu Chen, and Maria D. Llorente

CHAPTER 1 Selecting an Evidence-Based Practice 1
Patricia A. Areán and Amber Gum

Step 1: Identifying the Target Population 3
Step 2: Researching EBPs 3
Step 3: Deciding on the EBP 9
Step 4: Determining What to Do if No EBP Exists 13

CHAPTER 2 Assessing Feasibility 17
Jane E. Fisher, Claudia Drossel,
Michael A. Cucciare, and Craig Yury

Assessing Readiness 17
Measuring Organizational Readiness: 18
 A Review of the Literature
Assessing Organizational Climate for EBPs 21
Assessing Costs as the Bottom Line 22
Modifying and Implementing an Identified EBP 27
Maintaining Awareness of New EBPs 32

CHAPTER 3   Quality Management in Evidence-Based   37
             Service Programs
             Hongtu Chen, Rodolfo Vega, JoAnn E. Kirchner,
             James Maxwell, and Sue E. Levkoff

             Administrative Strategies for Quality Management   38
             Evaluation Strategies for Quality Management   56
             Discussion   63

CHAPTER 4   Culturally Grounding Evidence-Based Practice   67
             Ramón Valle, Elizabeth Stadick, Jane Latané, Virginia
             Cappeller, Monica de La Cerda, and Gregory Archer

             The Conceptual Base   67
             Program Experiences and Outcomes: 75
                Applying the CG EBP Framework
             Implementation, Documentation, Measurement,   84
                and Outcome Issues
             Lessons Learned and the Distance Yet to Go   91

CHAPTER 5   Evidence-Based Practices for the Assessment and   99
             Treatment of Depression, Anxiety, and Substance
             Use Disorders
             Jane E. Fisher, Michael A. Cucciare, Claudia Droßel, and
             Craig Yury

             Depression in Older Adults   99
             Anxiety in Older Adults   108
             Substance Use Disorders in Older Adults   118

CHAPTER 6   Evidence-Based Practices for Dementia and   135
             Schizophrenia
             Jane E. Fisher, Kyle E. Ferguson, and Claudia Droßel

             Dementia   135
             Schizophrenia in Late Life   146

CHAPTER 7   Evidence-Based Practices by Service Delivery   159
             Process
             Jeffrey A. Buchanan and Tiffany Berg

             Screening and Assessment   160
             Treatment   164
             Prevention and Outreach   172
             Discussion and Conclusions   174

CHAPTER 8 Evidence-Based Practices Within Special Settings   179
John M. Worrall, Stacey Cherup, Ruth A. Gentry,
Jane E. Fisher, and Hillary LeRoux

Faith-Based Organizations   179
Primary Care   181
Extended Care Settings   192
Services to Older Adults in Rural Communities   197

CHAPTER 9 Moving Toward Sustainable Services   209
Dean D. Krahn and Sue E. Levkoff

Should a Program Be Sustained?   209
What Makes Change More Likely to   210
    Be Sustained?
Defining Sustainability   211
Implications of the Literature   213
From Implementing to Sustaining a Program   215
Efforts to Sustain the Kajsiab House Project   217
Tips for Creating a Program That Is Sustainable   221
One Last View of Sustainability   223
Epilogue   224

Index   225

Contributors

Gregory Archer, PsyD, Program Evaluator, Tiempo de Oro Program, Valle del Sol Inc., Phoenix, AZ.

Patricia A. Areán, PhD, Associate Professor, Department of Psychiatry, University of California-San Francisco, CA.

Tiffany Berg, BS, Department of Psychology, Minnesota State University, Mankato, MN.

Jeffrey A. Buchanan, PhD, Assistant Professor of Psychology, Center on Aging, Minnesota State University, Mankato, MN.

Virginia Cappeller, PhD, Clinical Director, Health Improvement Program, Jewish Family and Children's Services, Tucson, AZ.

Monica de La Cerda, MEd, Principal Investigator, Tiempo de Oro Program, Valle del Sol Inc., Phoenix, AZ.

Stacey Cherup, BA, Department of Psychology, University of Nevada, Reno, NV.

Michael A. Cucciare, MA, Department of Psychology, University of Nevada, Reno, NV.

Claudia Droßel, PhD, Department of Psychology, University of Nevada, Reno, NV.

Kyle E. Ferguson, MA, Department of Psychology, University of Nevada, Reno, NV.

Ruth A. Gentry, MA, Department of Psychology, University of Nevada, Reno, NV.

Amber Gum, PhD, Florida Institute of Mental Health, University of South Florida, Tampa, FL.

JoAnn E. Kirchner, MD, Associate Director for Clinical Care, VA South Central, Mental Illness Research, Education, and Clinical Center (MIRECC); Associate Professor of Psychiatry, University of Arkansas for Medical Sciences, Little Rock, AR.

Dean D. Krahn, MD, MS, Clinical Associate Professor of Psychiatry, University of Wisconsin Medical School; Chief, Mental Health Service, William S. Middleton Memorial Veterans Hospital, Madison, WI.

Jane Latané, MEd, Program Coordinator, Health Improvement Program, Jewish Family and Children's Services Inc., Tucson, AZ.

Hillary LeRoux, BA, Department of Psychology, University of Nevada, Reno, NV.

Maria D. Llorente, MD, Director, Geriatric Psychiatry, Veterans Administration Medical Center; Associate Professor of Psychiatry, University of Miami School of Medicine, Miami, FL.

James Maxwell, PhD, Director of Health Policy and Management Research, John Snow Research & Training Institute, Inc., Boston, MA.

Elizabeth Stadick, BA, Coordinator, Tiempo de Oro Program, Valle del Sol, Inc., Phoenix, AZ.

Ramón Valle, PhD, Professor Emeritus, San Diego State University; Director, Alzheimer's Cross Cultural Research and Development (ACCORD), San Diego, CA.

Rodolfo Vega, PhD, Senior Consultant, Program Evaluation Specialist, John Snow Research & Training Institute, Inc., Boston, MA.

John M. Worrall, MBA, Department of Psychology, University of Nevada, Reno, NV.

Craig Yury, MA, Department of Psychology, University of Nevada, Reno, NV.

Foreword

One thing is sure. We have to do something. We have to do the best we know how at the moment . . . ; If it doesn't turn out right, we can modify it as we go along.

—*Franklin D. Roosevelt*

The pursuit of happiness is enshrined in the Declaration of Independence as one of our inalienable rights, but for too many older Americans the promise of the golden years is replaced by the reality of blue years. Positive aging in older Americans relies heavily on access to and receipt of quality and effective mental health services. Frequently, however, the mental health needs of our older neighbors, family members, and friends go unmet. As highlighted in the Positive Aging Act, first introduced in Congress on July 9, 2002, we must "adopt and implement evidence-based protocols, to the extent available, for prevalent mental health disorders" among seniors in our communities.

The good news is that in the past decade if we are to close this care gap, the research community has made tremendous progress in consolidating scientific evidence and expert consensus on processes for managing care for older adults with mental illnesses. The overall message is hopeful: (a) systematic screening can help successfully identify prevalent mental health problems in older persons and (b) there are scientifically proven ways to alleviate mental health problems such as depression and anxiety in older adults. These problems do not have to be part of the normal aging process. Our challenge is to translate this knowledge into practice, into everyday service delivery to older people and their families.

Most of the successful mental health service programs for older adults require integration and collaboration between mental health services and other medical and social services. The implementation of these evidence-based practices is challenging because it requires changes at many levels, including various service providers' behavior, organizational arrangements, and, most of all, the way we think about the problems and develop solutions. As with all worthy causes, making a change in the real world and turning a good idea into a good program take two sets of qualities and resources working in tandem. First, they take leadership, championing of changes, individual initiative, visionary thinking, determination, and a deep sense of social responsibility to start something worthwhile and overcoming inertia and the barriers that will inevitably arise. Second, they require cooperation, collaboration, peer support, teamwork, generosity, and collective wisdom and knowledge to get something completed.

With this observation in mind, I applaud *Evidence-Based Behavioral Health Practices for Older Adults: A Guide to Implementation*, as it will help people nurture and develop the skills necessary to try something new and innovative and to deliver better and more effective care to those in need. This book comes from a group of thoughtful people who have helped, observed, and researched the difficult and complicated process of implementing evidence-based mental health services for older Americans. I hope this book will bring about more learning and action among all of us involved in the cause of helping millions of older Americans live a positive and better life, the life they deserve.

Congressman Patrick J. Kennedy

Acknowledgments

We wish to express our gratitude to the many people who have directly or indirectly helped us in the production of this book. Most of all, we want to thank those frontline service leaders and developers of the Targeted Capacity Expansion (TCE) Programs designed to improve behavioral health programs for older adults. The thoughtfulness, diligence, and creativity of these program implementers are the inspiration for this book. It is their experience with the difficulties and their courage to overcome the barriers confronting them that made us realize the need for such a book. If those who are funded and supported need such a book, then many others who want to develop similar service programs for older adults will likely benefit from it as well. Since each TCE program involves many people, some of whom have already left their organizations, we want to acknowledge their contribution by mentioning the names of the participating organizations: La Clinica Del Pueblo in Washington, DC; COTTAGE Expanded Elder Services in Tucson, Arizona; ElderLynk Expansion Program in Kirksville, Missouri; Health Improvement in Tucson, Arizona; Kajsiab House in Madison, Wisconsin; Project FOCUS in El Paso, Texas; Senior Behavioral Health Service Program in San Francisco, California; Senior Outreach Program in Rochester, New York; and Tiempo de Oro Program in Phoenix, Arizona. A description of these programs can be found at www.positiveaging.org.

Our funding agency, the Center for Mental Health Services of the Substance Abuse and Mental Health Services Administration (SAMHSA), deserves our salute. Its original vision and continuous support along the way were critical to the success of the TCE Project. Our special thanks go to Betsy McDonel Herr, PhD, the project officer of the TCE program, and Neal Brown, MPA, chief of the Community Support Program at SAMHSA's Center for Mental Health Services, for their support, advice, and many technical contributions to the project.

We would also like to thank all of the older adults and their families participating in the services programs. Their presence, feedback, and guidance significantly enhanced and directed our efforts to improve care. They are the sustaining power and the ultimate justification for the meaning and value of our work.

We thank the many consultants for their thoughtful support for the service program developed at each site, and for those who participated in the initial teleconference meetings to help conceptualize this book.

We are grateful to Milly Krakow who provided important editorial support with her extraordinarily perceptive and helpful comments.

Introduction

Sue E. Levkoff, Hongtu Chen, and Maria D. Llorente

American health-care delivery systems are working to improve health services through research on and implementation of evidence-based practices (EBPs). Research on EBP has gained momentum since its inception almost a decade ago, but the service delivery field is increasingly challenged by the lack of guidance on processes for successfully implementing EBPs. This book provides critically needed guidance for behavioral health-care providers regarding the implementation of evidence-based practices to improve service delivery.

This book supports the nationwide effort to improve services for older Americans in response to the expansion of the aging population and the increasing demand for cost-effective mental health care of older persons. To improve the capacity and quality of mental health care for older adults, the nation must gather the available resources and equip its frontline service leaders and providers with adequate knowledge, training, and instruments for them to make urgently needed changes. Through our work with the Substance Abuse and Mental Health Services Administration (SAMHSA), a federal agency devoted to the improvement of mental health-care quality, we, as a group affiliated with the Positive Aging Resource Center (PARC) and its partner service sites, have learned many lessons about how to successfully implement evidence-based programs and principles in real-world clinical service settings. This book provides information on these lessons and on resources for frontline service providers.

COMPLEXITY OF EBP IMPLEMENTATION

Evidence-based practice is a conscious effort to use the best available evidence to guide decision making in the delivery of health services. It incorporates research findings and professional judgment and knowledge with individual patient characteristics and preferences in formulating clinical decisions (Dubouloz et al., 1999; Gerrish & Clayton, 2004; Goldman, Thelander, & Cleas-Goran, 2000). When implementing any EBP, one typically would consider following basic strategies:

- Integrating *research* with practice: use of current best evidence from relevant, valid research about the effects of different forms of health care (O'Rourke, 1997); systematically find, appraise, and use research findings as a basis for clinical decisions (Lockett, 1997).
- Including *evaluation* in practice: systematic application of rigorous scientific methods to the evaluation of the effectiveness of health-care interventions; an approach that promotes the collection, interpretation, and integration of valid, important and applicable patient-reported, clinician-observed, and research-derived evidence (McKibbon, 1998).
- Incorporating *clinical expertise*: integration of individual clinical expertise with the best available external clinical evidence from systematic research (Sackett, Rosenberg, Gray, Haynes, & Richardson, 1996; Bartels et al., 2002).
- Assessing *patient characteristics*: consideration of patient circumstances and preferences when assessing the interaction between the clinician and the client in order to improve the quality of clinical judgments (McKibbon, 1998).

Moving an EBP discussion from an academic setting to a clinical health-care setting is challenging and complex for several reasons. First, different organizations developing an EBP have different starting points, particularly with regard to cultural background, familiarity with types of evidence, ability to manage information and conduct evaluations, attitudes toward change and improving quality of services, and the ongoing daily functioning of the current program. Second, program planners may have different aims in mind: Some want to develop a program focusing only on outreach, prevention, screening, or treatment; others want to provide care for a population and community with a unique cultural profile.

Contextual variation may influence EBP implementers to take different routes in developing an evidence-based method or approach. Some may try to improve practice based on the *best scientific evidence* available, using their access to well-established EBP guidelines or protocols to fit to the site's service situation. Others may aim to improve practice by making conscious decisions based on *best available evidence*, especially in those circumstances where (a) it is difficult to find an established EBP guideline appropriate for a specific situation, or (b) there is a need to undertake a more innovative and groundbreaking experience-based approach in order to develop the service. Regardless of the approach, EBP implementation becomes part of a continuous quality improvement process, with an emphasis on translating, adapting, and integrating different levels of evidence and knowledge obtained from both scientific research and practice experience.

While handling the day-to-day tasks of developing a behavioral health clinical program, the EBP program administrators often need to address complicated issues related to resources development and constraints. To introduce changes necessary for an EBP implementation, the implementation leaders need to gain support from senior managers, form a coalition with service providers, and ask for extra effort from staff members. Developing an evidence-based behavioral health program for older adults often requires collaboration with other health or social service organizations, or at least integration of services among different departments within the same organizations. In addition, a community-based organization often has to seek external technical support and resources to help identify EBP guidelines, design program evaluation plans, and collect and analyze data or evidence to inform and justify major implementation decisions. Those who begin a program or intervention using the best scientific evidence available will have to incorporate new knowledge gained from local practice in particular settings. Similarly, those who begin with evidence derived from local practice and consensus based on expert opinion often need to develop more generalizable knowledge through efforts such as advanced program evaluation.

THE SYSTEM APPROACH TO A SUCCESSFUL EBP IMPLEMENTATION

The system approach is critical to the successful implementation of an EBP in mental health services (Berwick, 2002; Eddy 2005). This approach emphasizes the need to be aware of the service environment including the organizational and community setting, and the client's and provider's cultural context—before and during implementation of an EBP program. This system approach can be summarized into five operational principles that support the successful implementation of an EBP. These principles are further elaborated on in Chapters 1 through 4 and 9.

Principle 1—Selecting the best EBP with the best fit for the target population and service staff. The best EBP is not only based on those with the most rigorous scientific evidence: it should also be acceptable to and feasible for the consumer base and staff capability. The authors of Chapter 1 provide a logic model for identifying the most useful and promising EBP for the community.

Principle 2—Assessing feasibility for implementing an EBP with the whole journey in mind. Assessing the feasibility of implementing an EBP is not only about examining the readiness of the parent organization but also about broader issues. Strategies provided in Chapter 2 encourage the EBP implementers to augment information on clinical effectiveness and to look further ahead by assessing resources for training and maintenance of the project, barriers to implementation, and the degree to which the EBP should be modified in order to be applicable to a particular setting.

Principle 3—Managing quality of EBP implementation through involvement of people and evaluation of the entire organization. The success of program development depends on the project team's ability to utilize both human and information resources to orchestrate a thoughtful and persistent process of continuous improvement and assurance of the quality of implementation. Based on fundamental principles developed from the quality management movement since the 1950s, Chapter 3 provides recommendations for how to use the quality management process in developing an EBP program.

Principle 4—Developing EBP in a cultural context. Implementing an EBP requires integration of EBP principles with the cultural characteristics of both the client population and the service providers. A culturally grounded model for the application of evidence-based practice in mental and behavioral health is described in Chapter 4.

Principle 5—Sustaining an EBP program through thoughtful planning that ensures the EBP is embedded organically in its parent organization. To increase the likelihood of sustainability, the authors of Chapter 9 suggest that future mental health improvement projects must not only improve people's lives but must also positively impact the organization and community in which the project "lives."

In a review of all major studies of quality improvement work in health care in the past decades, Shojania and Grimshaw (2005) identified the success of any EBP effort as dependent on the implementers being willing to seek a comprehensive understanding of the problem. In the system approach, understanding the problem is mainly about understanding the specific *context* of the problem. To facilitate a consideration of the service context, Chapters 5 to 8 present information on how EBPs are practiced in relation to specific mental health conditions, service delivery processes, and service institutions.

The EBP implementation that uses a systems approach should keep the system, however defined, as an *open* system, to increase its chances to stay healthy, self-motivated, and essentially *good*. It is open to better services that should eventually benefit all parties involved (it is good); it is open to complexities intrinsically imbedded in the cultural context of service populations, organizational politics, and provider styles (it is good for whom, by whom); it is open to changes that should happen in a gradual, coordinated, and thoughtful manner (how it becomes good); and it is open to the future with sophisticated and flexible plans for sustainable services (how the good will last).

HOW TO USE THIS BOOK

We developed *Evidence-Based Behavioral Health Practices for Older Adults: A Guide to Implementation* as part of our efforts to improve the quality of mental health services for older adults and their families. This book was mostly written by faculty and coaches affiliated with the Positive Aging Resource Center (PARC) and its partner sites across the country. Although the content of this book is relevant to all people who work with elderly clients with mental-health needs, the following three groups of readers may find this how-to book particularly useful: (1) program administrators and clinical supervisors such as directors of mental-health programs, senior centers, nursing homes, and senior day-care programs; (2) health-care professionals in both the fields of mental health services and geriatric services, including clinical social workers, nurses, psychiatrists, psychologists, occupational therapists, physical therapists, nutritionists, and recreational therapists; and (3) teachers and students participating in courses related to service delivery, service program development, health administration, aging, mental health, and rehabilitation. The first two groups will find this book useful and beneficial in helping them move an innovative idea to a real and sustainable improvement in a service program. This book will provide the third group with an in-depth understanding of one of the critical challenges in the health-care field: how to improve quality of health care through evidence-based practice.

Evidence-Based Behavioral Health Practices for Older Adults: A Guide to Implementation can also serve as a reference for evidence-based geriatric behavioral health materials, and the implementation of these materials. Along with our online information on EBPs in geriatric mental health care (www.positiveaging.org) and the references cited at the end of each chapter, we hope this book will become a useful tool and resource for all those who care about and provide services to older adults.

REFERENCES

Bartels, S. J., Dums, A. R., Oxman, T. E., Schneider, L. S., Areán, P. A., Alexopoulus, G. S., et al. (2002). Evidence-based practices in geriatric mental health care. *Psychiatric Services, 53,* 1419–1431.

Berwick, D. M. (2002). A user's manual for the IOM's "Quality Chasm" report. *Health Affairs, 21*(3), 80–90.

Capra, F. (1996). *The web of life: The new scientific understanding of living systems.* New York: Anchor Books.

Dubouloz, C. J., Egan, M., Vallerand, J., VonZweck, C. (1999). Occupational therapists' perceptions of evidence-based practice. *American Journal of Occupational Therapy 53*(5), 445–453.

Eddy, D. M. (2005). Evidence-based medicine: A unified approach. *Health Affairs, 24,* 9–17.

Gerrish, K., & Clayton, J. (2004). Promoting evidence-based practice: An organizational approach. *Journal of Nursing Management, 12,* 114–123.

Goldman, H. H., Thelander, S., & Cleas-Goran, W. (2000). Organizing mental health services: An evidence-based approach. *Journal of Mental Health Policy and Economics, 3,* 69–75.

Lockett, T. (1997). *Evidence-based and cost effective medicine for the uninitiated.* Oxford, New York: Radcliffe Medical Press.

McKibbon, K. A. (1998). Evidence-based practice. *Bulletin of the Medical Library Association, 86*(3), 396–401.

O'Rourke, P. J. (1997). Endpiece: Escaping the future. *British Medical Journal, 315*(7118), 1282.

Sackett, D. L., Rosenberg, W. M. C., Gray, J. M., Haynes, R. B., & Richardson, W. S. (1996). Evidence-based medicine: What it is and what it isn't. *British Medical Journal, 321,* 71–72.

Shojania, K. G., & Grimshaw, J. M. (2005). Evidence-based quality improvement: The state of the science. *Health Affairs, 24*(1), 138–150.

CHAPTER 1

Selecting an Evidence-Based Practice

Patricia A. Areán and Amber Gum

Several states and counties in the United States have specific governmental mandates to ensure that mental health providers who work in public mental health settings provide evidence-based practices (EBP). For example, California's Proposition 63 "Millionaire Tax" specifically provides funding to county mental health providers contingent on their provision of evidence-based practices. However, there has been very little guidance for mental health providers regarding processes and techniques for identifying those practices.

Identifying an EBP requires time and dedication. Breaking the process down into steps makes this daunting task more manageable. These steps include (1) identifying the target population, (2) researching EBPs for the target population, (3) deciding on the EBP, and (4) determining what to do if no EBP exists. In some situations, there will be no EBP at all; programs can either modify an EBP, or employ an *emerging practice* (EP, an intervention with some research support but not to the degree of an EBP) or a *service-informed practice* (SIP, an intervention widely and uniformly used in the community but having no scientific evidence base).

The purpose of this chapter is to detail how to implement these four steps. It can serve as a guide to community mental health programs searching for the best EBP for their community. See Figure 1.1 for a logic model to use in making decisions about an EBP selection.

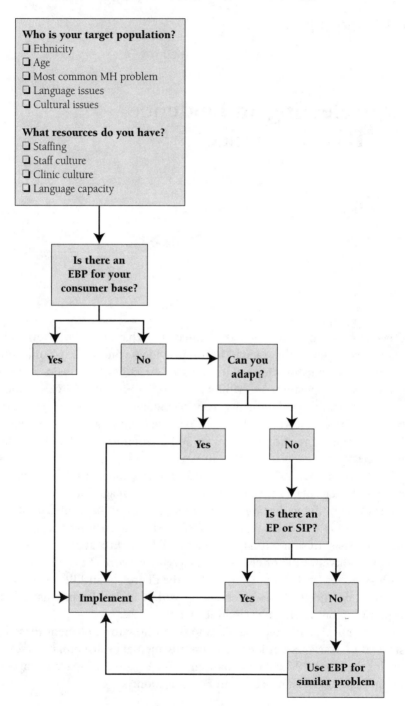

FIGURE 1.1   Logic model for EBP selection.

STEP 1: IDENTIFYING THE TARGET POPULATION

The first step in the process is to identify the target community. This step involves obtaining answers to the following questions: Which disorder is most common in your setting? Does your clinic represent mostly one minority group or is the clinic population diverse? Who are the staff members in the clinic and what skills do they possess?

CASE STUDY

To illustrate how selecting an evidence-based practice works, we discuss our experience in moving EBPs for depression and agitation management to assisted living facilities. Our first step was to conduct a survey of needs that facility managers and frontline staff faced in working with their consumers. Our survey of more than 400 facilities in three northern California counties found facility managers wanted help with agitation management and depression. We then identified EBPs (based on the method described in Step 2) and presented the treatments to staff and managers in focus group settings to determine their interest, the fit of these models with their clientele, and the capabilities of the staff to implement these EBPs. Based on feedback from the groups, we determined that (1) the interventions needed to be adapted culturally, not only for the clients, but also for the staff providing them (many staff in assisted living facilities were monolingual, speaking Tagalog and Spanish); (2) some EBPs needed to be delivered by outside professionals, while others could be delivered by existing staff; and (3) there would be a need for ongoing consultation as the new EBPs were implemented in these settings. This information helped in the selection of the best EBPs and the best model of dissemination.

(continues later in the chapter)

STEP 2: RESEARCHING EBPS

The second step is to conduct comprehensive research on the target problem and the EBPs that address the problem. This step involves reviewing the literature and developing an understanding of the details of the EBP. Researching EBPs requires time to go to the library, collect articles, sort information, and read through the details of the EBP. This step can at times be exciting as you learn more information about the target problem, and at other times frustrating as you discover how little there may be for your target population.

Phase 1: The Literature Search

Search engines or large databases are helpful in identifying research articles and literature reviews with information on EBPs for your target population. Academic databases are excellent resources for finding these reviews and articles. Abstracts of most professional mental health and substance abuse publications (i.e., articles on empirical research studies, journals, books, book chapters) about older adults are included in PubMed and PsycInfo, which are accessible online. PubMed includes all publications abstracted in the Medline database and is available to the public at no cost. PsycInfo is a product of the American Psychological Association and is available to the general public for a fee. University libraries generally offer free public access to these databases; several professional organizations also provide access to these databases for their members.

PubMed and PsycInfo hold virtually all of the abstracts for research publications relevant to aging and mental health. In addition to empirical research studies, these databases also include literature reviews of journals, books, and book chapters. Literature reviews are an excellent place to start reading in a topic area, particularly for large topics for which it would be too time-consuming to read each research article (e.g., late-life depression). The primary benefit of searching these academic databases is the quality of publications. Journal articles included in these databases undergo a rigorous peer review process before being accepted for publication. Books and book chapters also usually go through a peer review process or at least an intensive peer-editing process. Another important benefit of using these databases is that all publications are catalogued by a variety of keywords, methodologies, and publication type, simplifying the document search. Finally, these databases allow users to set up searches that can be repeated at regular intervals and that will automatically e-mail the new publications that meet the search criteria. Likewise, many professional journals now offer *e-TOCs* (table of contents), in which users can sign up via the journal's Web site to receive the table of contents through e-mail whenever a new issue is released.

Most libraries throughout the United States provide tutorials on literature search methods. The most fruitful place to start your search is to use *keywords*, or general words that describe what you are looking for. For example, if you are interested in looking for evidence-based treatment for late life depression, common keywords to use are "depression," "late-life," "treatments," and "geriatric." It may take time to find the right keywords. If you are interested in treatment for Hispanic populations, you may have to use a variety of terms to get all the available information. For instance, in addition to "Hispanic," you may also have to use the terms "Latino," "Mexican,"

"Cuban," and "Puerto Rican" to get all the papers there are on the general Hispanic community. You can narrow your search by listing only recent articles by specifying years of publication. In PsycInfo, you can also limit the search to review articles, articles, or books.

Phase 2: Learning More About the EBP

Once existing EBPs for the target population have been identified, the second phase in this step involves locating the toolkits, guidelines, or manuals that describe the EBP in detail in order to make an informed decision among the available choices. *Toolkits* consist of instructions regarding the latest treatment for a mental health problem and provide tools to implement EBPs, including assessment tools for identifying the target problem, patient information materials regarding the problem, algorithms for medication management, and manuals for providing psychosocial interventions. The MacArthur Depression in Primary Care Tool Kit (www.depression-primarycare.org/clinicians/toolkits/) and the Substance Abuse and Mental Health Service Agency (SAMHSA) toolkits (http://mentalhealth.samhsa.gov/cmhs/communitysupport/toolkits.asp) are good examples of online toolkits. *Guidelines* are typically for medication management methods for mental health problems and include information on dosing and side effects for first- and second-line medications, how to decide on which medication to use, how the medication should be introduced (e.g., slowly), the time line for response, how often the provider should monitor side effects and symptom profiles, and when to change doses or medications. *Manuals* are typically guidelines for psychosocial interventions, and the theory behind the intervention, including step-by-step information about how to deliver the intervention. Most toolkits, guidelines, and manuals can be located easily online and are often available for free.

Online Resources

The most trusted sources of online information are government-sponsored Web sites, national and international organizations, and academic institutions. When reading online information, consider the source of the information and its consistency with other information and general research and clinical principles. New resources are regularly added or upgraded online, making it important to regularly update searches.

Government agencies provide relevant information online in order to facilitate dissemination of knowledge and implementation of EBPs. SAMHSA's Web site contains a range of online information and offers many publications and treatment improvement protocols free of charge through its clearinghouses. For example, the SAMHSA Web site includes several treatment improvement protocols for substance abuse treatment, including a protocol tailored for older adults.

The Positive Aging Resource Center (PARC) was created in 2002 by a SAMHSA initiative to improve quality and access to mental health services for older adults. PARC provides information for older adults and their caregivers, health and social service providers, and policymakers. The section of the Web site for professionals (e.g., www.positiveaging.org) includes information on opportunities to connect with other professionals, training procedures, EBPs, assessment tools, and funding opportunities.

Other government agencies and professional organizations provide information about aging and mental health (National Institute of Mental Health at www.nimh.gov; National Institute on Aging at www.nia.gov). However, while much of this information is useful for consumers, the information for professionals is fairly general, with few details on specific EBPs. Similarly, professional organizations make available mental health information on their Web sites, some of which is specific to older adults, such as the American Association for Geriatric Psychiatry (www.aagp.org), International Psychogeriatric Association (www.ipa-online.org), American Psychiatric Association (www.psych.org), and American Psychological Association (www.apa.org). Organizations that focus on diseases common in late life also have useful information, such as the Alzheimer's Association or American Heart Association.

Some researchers and clinicians post information about EBPs on their institution's Web sites or create their own Web sites. One example is the Stanford Older Adult and Family Center (http://www.med.stanford.edu/oac/), which provides treatment protocols for psychosocial interventions for caregivers of older adults with dementia. Another example is the IMPACT (Improving Mood-Promoting Access to Collaborative Treatment) Web site (www.impact.ucla.edu), which provides links for researchers and clinicians to acquire training and resources on the IMPACT model of comprehensive care for late-life depression in primary care settings (Unützer et al., 2002). For many funded research studies, the results and information on how to access additional information are posted on the Web site of the funding agency.

Conferences and Professional Organizations

One of the main purposes of professional organizations and conferences is to provide a forum for sharing developments with colleagues. Research presentations, roundtable discussions, and informal social hours are all vehicles for networking with other professionals in the field and for sharing information about promising new practices. Additionally, many conferences offer workshops for clinicians to further develop specific skills. In the United States, national annual conferences with information specific to aging and mental health include the Gerontological Society of America, joint American Society on Aging/National Council on the Aging, and American Association of Geriatric Psychiatry. Other mental health and social service conferences often have some aging-related presentations. Regional conferences are often a productive forum for local networking opportunities. For example, the annual meeting of the Florida Coalition on Mental Health and Aging, one of several state coalition conferences, draws researchers, policymakers, clinicians of various backgrounds, and consumers. The Web site of the National Coalition on Mental Health and Aging (www.ncoa.org) includes links to local and state-level aging and mental health coalitions. Many organizations offer other resources for learning about best practices, including online materials for members only, directories, workshops, continuing education opportunities, and Listserve capabilities (whereby members can e-mail the entire body of members).

Personal Consultation

Contacting the authors of publications that look promising is another method for obtaining information. Being available for correspondence with interested readers is a responsibility of authors who publish peer-reviewed journal articles; their contact information should be available in the article and on their university or organization's Web site. Although it can be intimidating the first time you contact someone, you will find that most people are quite friendly and helpful. They are glad that someone is interested in their work and want to see effective methods be applied more widely. Some authors will want information about your setting and may require some training for you or your staff to use their protocols; most authors will provide direction toward resources for training and implementation.

Local colleagues in clinical or academic settings can be a resource for assistance in identifying EBPs. When consulting with someone, particularly if you do not have funds to pay consultation fees, consider other ways in which you could collaborate or help their professional efforts. For example, you might consult a local psychology professor on EBPs for suicide screening in primary care, while allowing her to develop empirical research methods to evaluate the success of your program or develop other research projects in your setting.

See Table 1.1 for selected Internet sources for information on aging and mental health.

TABLE 1.1   Selected Internet Sources for Information on Aging and Mental Health

Organization	Internet Address (http://)
Scientific Databases	
PubMed	pubmed.gov (free public access)
PsycInfo	www.apa.org/psycinfo (available for free at most university libraries, fees apply for general public access)
EBPs, Treatment Guidelines	
Substance Abuse and Mental Health Services Administration (SAMHSA)	www.samhsa.gov
Positive Aging Resource Center (PARC)	www.positiveaging.org
Sample Researcher-Initiated EBP Web Sites	
Stanford Older Adult and Family Center	www.med.stanford.edu/oac
IMPACT Depression Care Program	impact.ucla.edu
Mental Health Information	
National Institute of Mental Health (NIMH)	www.nimh.nih.gov
	www.nimh.nih.gov/HealthInformation/depoldermenu.cfm
American Association for Geriatric Psychiatry (AAGP)	www.aagpgpa.org
American Psychiatric Association (APA)	www.psych.org
American Psychological Association (APA)	www.apa.org
	www.geropsych.org (clinical geropsychology section)
	apadiv20.phhp.ufl.edu (aging division)
International Psychogeriatric Association (IPA)	www.ipa-online.org
Aging Information	
Administration on Aging	www.aoa.dhhs.gov/
Alzheimer's Association	www.alz.org/
American Society on Aging	www.asaging.org/
Gerontological Society of America	www.geron.org
National Council on the Aging	www.ncoa.org/
National Institute on Aging (NIA)	www.nia.nih.gov
Advocacy Organizations, Coalitions	
National Coalition on Mental Health and Aging	www.ncmha.org
	www.ncmha.org/coalitions.php3 (state coalitions)

STEP 3: DECIDING ON THE EBP

When gathering information about various practices that address the target population and treatment, it is important to consider the criteria by which to evaluate and choose among them. These criteria include the empirical evidence, as well as the cultural, social, and functional context of the patient population and setting (see Fig. 1.2).

Evaluating the Empirical Evidence

The premise of the EBP movement is to improve the quality of health care by applying those practices that have the strongest empirical support. There are two broad questions to consider when evaluating research studies: (1) Is there strong evidence that the treatment (as opposed to other variables) caused the improvements? and (2) How are the findings likely to generalize to the target population, problems, and setting? Evaluating the evidence of the treatment impact uses criteria detailed in Chapter 2 (Assessing Feasibility). The number and quality of randomized clinical trials will help determine if the practice is an EBP.

To evaluate the generalizability of the findings, consider factors such as the characteristics of the study sample in relation to the target population, including diagnostic category, age, sex, race/ethnicity, education, income level, rural or urban setting, and residential or medical setting. Research studies frequently have more homogenous participants than are found in typical clinical settings. For example, most studies of late-life depression have focused on major depressive disorder (MDD). Subthreshold forms of depression are more common in older adults across clinical settings, however, and still cause significant functional impairment (Lewinsohn, Solomon, Seeley, & Zeiss, 2000). Likewise, researchers historically have experienced difficulties enrolling sufficient numbers of racial and ethnic minority elders into clinical research (Areán & Gallagher-Thompson, 1996). Fortunately, recent advances have been made in terms of researching treatments for a wider range of diagnostic categories and diverse samples.

Consider the Context of the Setting and Population

A certain EBP may work well in a study, but it may not be feasible in a specific real-world clinical setting or applicable with a specific population. Therefore, one must also consider the multifaceted context for applying the

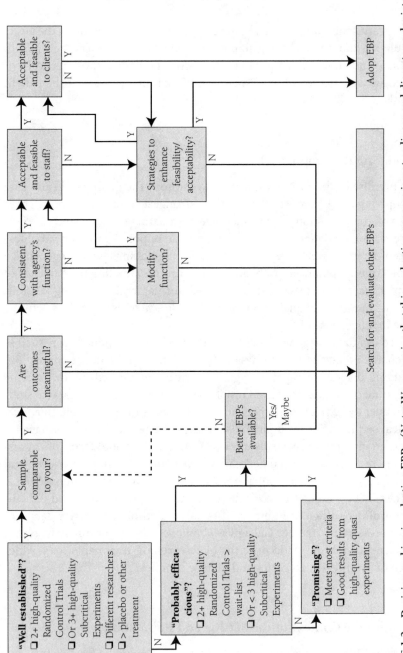

FIGURE 1.2   Decision making in selecting EBPs. (*Note:* We recognize that this evaluation process is not as linear and discrete as depicted in this figure, which is merely provided as a guide.)

EBP, including the culture of the work setting, feasibility issues, and the cultural and social aspects of the target population.

Functional Context of Setting

First, consider how EBP fits with the mission and priorities of the organization. For example, many primary care clinics do not consider extensive mental health or substance abuse treatment to be part of their mission. EBPs that might fit within their mission include screening and referral procedures. In contrast, some federally funded community clinics provide interdisciplinary care that addresses medical, psychological, and social needs of its low-income community-dwelling older adults. Therefore, in addition to a primary care component, these clinics often have a social services component that employs case managers, social workers, and a clinical psychologist. It is feasible, then, for these clinics to consider integrating actual treatments into their settings.

The culture of the work setting and staff attitudes are also very relevant in selecting EBPs. When deciding among EBPs with similar levels of empirical support, it is useful to consider whether one better matches the general work climate or staff preferences of a given organization. With sufficient training and resources, professionals from different frameworks can learn a variety of new protocols, but training is simplified when the EBP in question is acceptable to the staff and is closer to their usual approach. Although trained therapists learn problem-solving therapy very well, we have found that therapists with a cognitive-behavioral background find the new techniques to be a more natural fit with their usual approach. However, we caution against *only* using EBPs that closely align with staff's current approaches as professionals often do benefit from looking at clinical situations from a new perspective.

Feasibility Issues

A number of feasibility issues related to implementation need to be addressed. What kinds of specialists are needed to implement a certain EBP? What type of training is needed? How much time and physical space are needed with clients? What types of payment options are available? Other sections of this book discuss implementation issues in greater detail (Chapter 2, Assessing Feasibility), but it is important to consider the implementation process while evaluating potential EBPs. Obviously, those practices that require fewer resources, less time, and less specialized expertise will be more efficient to implement.

Cultural and Social Aspects of the Population

In examining the cultural and social aspects of the target population, one must ask: Will clients accept and participate in the service? For example, antidepressant medications are generally effective in treating late-life depression. However, several studies suggest that black adults are more likely to prefer and use psychotherapy and less likely to use antidepressant medications (Brown, Schulberg, Sacco, Perel, & Houck, 1999; Cooper et al., 2003; Dwight-Johnson, Sherbourne, Liao, & Wells, 2000); therefore, in settings that serve large numbers of black older adults, offering EBPs such as psychotherapy will be more effective than offering antidepressant medications. Stigma and lack of knowledge often contribute to unwillingness to accept mental health services, and it is therefore important to consider the general attitudes of the target population and methods for enhancing acceptability.

Older adults face a number of barriers to engaging in services, such as finances, transportation, physical disability and illness, and other constraints on their time, such as caregiving. Thus, for each potential EBP, one should ask: What barriers will clients face trying to access this service? What steps can be taken to remove these barriers? Older adults are more likely to access mental health and substance abuse services if they are integrated into medical and social service settings (Bartels et al., 2004). Generally, EBPs that are more portable, require fewer client responsibilities, have sufficient funding, and accommodate physical disability or illness will result in greater access and utilization.

CASE STUDY

(continued)

As described in Step 1, when we employed Step 3 for our assisted living project, we had to consider several factors. For each target disorder, we had EBPs that required training and resources that many of the facility staff did not have; we had to fit the EBP concepts into the cultural understanding of the frontline staff. We also found that no two facilities were alike. For instance, some facilities were corporately owned and housed a large number of beds, with different staffing layers (physicians or nurses), while others were family owned, having a small number of bed units and only administrators and certified nursing assistants

(CNAs). Further, many of the CNAs did not speak English, an indication that training for an environmental intervention would be a challenge. We therefore created a model of implementing the EBPs that included training in depression and dementia that allowed for staff discussion of their conceptualization of these disorders, ongoing support from the training team, and buy-in from all levels of staff at the facilities.

(continues)

STEP 4: DETERMINING WHAT TO DO IF NO EBP EXISTS

In most circumstances, EBPs for mental health problems will not have a substantial evidence base for certain subpopulations, such as older adults with anxiety or older Asians with depression. The most common scenario is one in which an EBP exists for a disorder but has yet to be studied extensively in a certain demographic group. The next likely scenario is a situation in which there is not yet any evidence in support of existing treatments for a disorder, as in the case of medication management for agitation (Holden & Gitlesen, 2004). There are solutions for both these scenarios.

Existing EBP With No Evidence for a Target Demographic Group

If there is an EBP that seems to be a good fit for a particular setting, but there is no evidence of its effectiveness with the target group, one should contact the creator of the EBP and inquire about any ongoing research of the EBP for the target demographic group. If there is no such research, one can ask the EBP creator to partner with the agency to adapt the intervention. For instance, an Asian-focused rehabilitation service for severely mentally ill wanted to employ an EBP for rehabilitation that had not been used with Asian populations. The agency contacted the EBP creator who agreed to assist in an adaptation of the model. This collaboration resulted in a fruitful partnership; the agency was able to obtain implementation guidance from an expert in the EBP and the expert was able to collect data to support a larger trial testing the model in Asian communities. If the creator of the EBP is not able to assist with an adaptation, a mental health clinician who has expertise working with the target group may be able to assist with the adaptation.

No EBP Exists

In those cases where no EBP exists, one may use either an emerging practice or an SIP (service informed practice). The method for identifying emerging best practices is similar to the methods for identifying EBPs. Identifying SIPs is more difficult. SIPs are often spread by word of mouth, and thus networking with other agencies that serve a similar population may yield a potentially useful SIP. In the event that none of these methods yield results, try to identify an EBP that targets a similar problem or population. For instance, if the target mental health issue is dysthymia and no EBP exists, using an EBP for major depression may be the next best intervention.

CASE STUDY

(continued)

To illustrate with our assisted living example, we identified all the research that had been done on treatment for depression and agitation in older adults with physical and cognitive impairments. We found that while the evidence base for psychotherapies in cognitive impaired adults was weak, there was a good evidence base for medication management for depression. Conversely, while there was no good evidence base for medication management of agitation, there was a solid evidence base for environmental interventions. Because we were committed to offering consumers both behavioral and medication treatment options for both mental health problems, we found that we would need to investigate further to find an alternative EBP for depression and to find medication alternatives for agitation.

Our struggle to find an evidence-based psychotherapy program for depression in late life and an evidence-based medication management program for agitation fell under this category. For the psychotherapy program, we decided to investigate emerging best practices that had potential for our population. We settled on one therapy that not only reported one very positive result for older adults with cognitive impairment and depression but was also an intervention that could be delivered by nonmental-health providers, fitting our desire to have nursing staff learn to manage depression behaviorally. The medication management for agitation posed a bigger challenge. By searching the National Institute of Mental Health Web site for funded studies on agitation management, we discovered that a multisite study was underway using a treatment algorithm that mirrored what was felt to be the best practice available for agitation. We were able to obtain the algorithm for our purposes.

In sum, identifying an EBP with the best fit for your staff and consumer base is a challenge. The most important step is a thoughtful consideration of the target population and the available resources. All steps following should flow naturally from your mission.

REFERENCES

Areán, P. A., & Gallagher-Thompson, D. (1996). Issues and recommendations for the recruitment and retention of older ethnic minority adults into clinical research. *Journal of Consulting and Clinical Psychology, 64,* 875–880.

Bartels, S. J., Coakley, E. H., Zubritsky, C., Ware, J. H., Miles, K. M., Areán, P. A., et al. (2004). Improving access to geriatric mental health services: A randomized trial comparing treatment engagement with integrated versus enhanced referral care for depression, anxiety, and at-risk alcohol use. *American Journal of Psychiatry, 161,* 1455–1462.

Brown, C., Schulberg, H. C., Sacco, D., Perel, J. M., & Houck, P. R. (1999). Effectiveness of treatments for major depression in primary medical practice: A post hoc analysis of outcomes for African American and white patients. *Journal of Affective Disorders, 53,* 185–192.

Cooper, L. A., Gonzales, J. J., Gallo, J. J., Rost, K. M., Meredith, L. S., Rubenstein, L. V., et al. (2003). The acceptability of treatment for depression among African-American, Hispanic, and white primary care patients. *Medical Care, 41,* 479–489.

Dwight-Johnson, M., Sherbourne, C. D., Liao, D., & Wells, K. B. (2000). Treatment preferences among depressed primary care patients. *Journal of General Internal Medicine, 15,* 527–534.

Holden, B., & Gitlesen, J. P. (2004). Psychotropic medication in adults with mental retardation: Prevalence, and prescription practices. *Research in Developmental Disabilities, 25*(6), 509–521.

Lewinsohn, P. M., Solomon, A., Seeley, J. R., & Zeiss, A. (2000). Clinical implications of "subthreshold" depressive symptoms. *Journal of Abnormal Psychology, 109,* 345–351.

Unützer, J., Katon, W., Callahan, C. M., Williams, J. W., Jr., Hunkeler, E., Harpole, L., et al. (2002). Collaborative care management of late-life depression in the primary care setting: A randomized controlled trial. *Journal of the American Medical Association, 288,* 2836–2845.

CHAPTER 2

Assessing Feasibility

Jane E. Fisher, Claudia Drossel, Michael A. Cucciare,
and Craig Yury

In this chapter, we focus on procedures for assessing an organization's readiness to implement evidence-based practices (EBPs). It is important to assess feasibility including the organizational climate for the EBP, costs of an EBP initiative, processes for modifying and implementing an identified EBP, and strategies for maintaining awareness of new EBPs.

ASSESSING READINESS

What is readiness assessment and why is it important when implementing EBPs? Readiness assessment involves thoroughly examining an organization's willingness and ability to adopt and implement an innovation (Poats & Salvaneschi, 2003). The term *implementation* refers to the transition period during which targeted health-care providers (i.e., those involved in direct service delivery) become increasingly skillful and committed to the use of EBPs (Klein & Sorra, 1996).

Measuring an organization's readiness for implementing an innovation such as an EBP requires that the organization methodically examine its existing cultural, structural, and technological characteristics. Readiness assessment may include surveying health-care providers regarding their attitudes toward adopting new approaches to treatment and assessing the extent to which existing information systems will conform to the requirements of implementing the EBP (e.g., data collection and quality improvement). A readiness assessment should provide a health-care organization with a preliminary understanding of the challenges it is likely to face when adopting and implementing EBPs (Poats & Salvaneschi, 2003).

What general factors should be considered? It is important for an organization considering the implementation of EBPs to first exam its readiness for change. Assessing readiness can reduce or prevent costly problems associated with implementation (Poats and Salvaneschi, 2003), and a high level of readiness to change is associated with increased chance of successful outcomes (Snyder-Halpern, 2001). Poats and Salvaneschi suggest that an organization first consider the following general questions:

- Are your organization's high-level executives committed to the implementation of EBPs?
- Is your organization prepared to budget a sufficient amount of funding to successfully implement EBPs?
- Is your health-care staff willing to devote a sufficient amount of time and effort to the implementation effort?
- Are your current health-care practices and organizational structure consistent with your organization's vision for the future?
- Are your health-care providers ready for a collaborative work environment?
- Have you clearly defined the service levels (e.g., community needs) that are required to support the use of evidence-based practices in your setting?

MEASURING ORGANIZATIONAL READINESS: A REVIEW OF THE LITERATURE

Organizational readiness characteristics that are associated with the successful adoption and implementation of EBPs include *cultural/organizational characteristics* and *staff characteristics* (Poats and Salvaneschi, 2003).

Cultural and Organizational Characteristics

Organizational readiness for implementing an innovation is considered the best predictor of employee commitment to that organization (Ingersoll, Kirsch, Merk, & Lightfoot, 2000). Readiness is evident when (a) all executive decision makers are highly committed to the implementation of EBPs; (b) all executive decision makers understand the financial and time commitments necessary to successfully implement EBPs and are committed to making these investments; (c) there is a consensus throughout the organization that implementing EBPs is consistent with the organization's goals (i.e., consistent with the goal of providing evidence-based treatments); and (d) health-care providers involved in service delivery support the implementation of EBPs and understand its value to patients (Ingersoll et al., 2000).

Cultural/organizational readiness is also evident in domains such as knowledge, resources, skills, values and goals, and implementation and maintenance readiness (Snyder-Halpern, 2001).

Knowledge Readiness

Knowledge readiness is the extent to which individuals (i.e., executive decision makers and health-care providers) involved in the implementation of EBPs understand the implementation issues. Knowledge readiness includes both general and specific knowledge. General knowledge readiness includes an organization's previous experiences with implementing innovations and addressing challenges that are likely to emerge for a specific organization during the implementation process (e.g., deficiencies in staff skill) and solutions to those challenges (e.g., additional training). Specific knowledge readiness includes an understanding of an organization's clinical practice standards (e.g., the organization's and providers' goals regarding treatment delivery) and the impact of those standards on treatment delivery and patient outcomes (Snyder-Halpern, 2001).

Staff Characteristics

Providers involved in direct service delivery must support the adoption of EBPs for implementation to be successful. Evidence of support (Stewart, 1994) includes

- Providers' affiliated with the organization and involved in direct patient care report that they believe that the adoption of EBPs will improve the treatment delivery (i.e., will result in beneficial outcomes for patients and be relatively easy to adopt and administer).
- Providers and executive decision makers perceive their relationship as collaborative and open.
- Providers are actively involved in the decisions regarding implementing EBPs into clinical practice.
- Providers have opportunities to participate actively in the implementation of EBPs by being directly responsible for key objectives, guiding the implementation team, and promoting the implementation to the community of providers in the organization.

Staff Skill Readiness

Staff skill readiness is determined through assessment of provider training history and skill level, previous experience with EBPs, perceptions of the benefits of administering EBPs, extent to which providers are satisfied with EBPs, degree of perceived and desired involvement in the implementation process, and extent to which providers are committed to the health-care organization (Snyder-Halpern, 2001).

Resource Readiness

According to Snyder-Halpern (2001), resource readiness refers to an organization's ability to support the implementation of EBPs. This readiness factor requires that administrators and health-care providers understand the types and availability of resources necessary to successfully implement EBPs. For example, the implementation of an EBP may require that health-care providers competently administer psychological treatments with which they are unfamiliar. An organization confronting this issue will need to either (a) provide training and, ideally, ongoing supervision to their providers in the delivery of the EBP or (b) hire health-care providers who can demonstrate proficiency in the administration of the EBP. If new training is the desired path, decisions regarding who will conduct the training (i.e., someone in-house or a consultant) will need to be addressed (Snyder-Halpern, 2001).

Resource readiness is also reflected in an organization's readiness for ongoing quality improvement (QI). Depending on the technical readiness of an organization (i.e., the ability of an organization's hardware and software to support implementation efforts), an organization interested in QI will need to purchase computer equipment and statistical software, conduct data collection (e.g., chart review), and have access to statistical consultants. Other factors such as finances and availability of space and clinical supervisors are considered part of resource readiness (Snyder-Halpern, 2001).

Values and Goals Readiness

Values and goals readiness (sometimes referred to as *gap analysis*) reflects the fit between an organization's preimplementation structural and non-structural characteristics and the characteristics of the relevant EBPs. Structural characteristics include the number of health-care providers and employees, type of health-care organization, the level of employee autonomy, formalization and specialization, and organizational goals. Nonstructural characteristics include the level of bureaucracy, management style, political climate, staff interdependence, and decision-making processes.

Implementation and Maintenance Readiness

The process of implementation and maintenance readiness consists of introducing EBPs to providers and examining whether providers and consumers find them acceptable. Behavioral indexes of successful adoption are evident when providers consistently and competently implement the EBP, adhere to the specific evidence-based protocols, and report a high degree of satisfaction (i.e., providers find the EBP effective and relatively easy to administer) (Drake et al., 2001).

ASSESSING ORGANIZATIONAL CLIMATE FOR EBPs

In their model of innovation implementation, Klein and Sorra (1996) argue that effective implementation of EBPs results from (a) an organizational climate (or culture) for change and (b) the fit between EBPs and the values of health-care providers involved in a health-care organization (i.e., innovation-values fit). Organizational climate refers to providers' perceptions about the use of EBPs and, in particular, the extent to which they feel the use of EBPs is rewarded, supported, and expected within the health-care organization. A high degree of organizational climate fosters the use of EBPs by empowering providing providers with the skills necessary to implement EBPs; making incentives available to providers who use EBPs and using disincentives when EBPs are not used (when appropriate); and, perhaps most important, removing any obstacles that may interfere with the use of EBPs. The following five factors will produce an optimal climate for EBP implementation:

1. Readily available training in the use of EBPs to ensure competency.
2. Ample time to learn EBPs.
3. Following initial training, access to ongoing supervision to ensure adherence to the EBPs.
4. Prompt response to provider concerns regarding the use of EBPs by those responsible for guiding the implementation process.
5. Routine monitoring and rewards provided by administrators for the use of EBPs.

Focusing solely on external incentives as a means of promoting provider compliance in using EBPs can affect the generalization and maintenance of the EBP. Klein and Sorra (1996) note that providers who perceive the use of EBPs only as a pathway to obtain rewards (e.g., monetary rewards or to gain authority within an organization) may be compliant but lack investment in EBPs. In contrast, providers who perceive the use of EBPs as consistent with their values (e.g., providing best practices to patients) are more likely to be invested and committed to using EBPs.

Innovation-values fit refers to the degree to which providers' values coincide with the use of EBPs. Poor fit occurs when policy issues such as providing the most cost-effective interventions to patients and having the requirement of documenting adherence to EBPs are the impetus for a health-care organization to implement EBPs (Goldman et al., 2001). These priorities often conflict with the values of health-care providers to provide quality services. Specific strategies for maximizing innovation-values fit among target health-care providers include (see Mueser, Torrey, Lynde, Singer, & Drake, 2003):

- Administrator should attempt to address the needs and concerns of target providers by conducting focus groups. Focus groups can be conducted for all target providers (e.g., case managers, psychiatrists, psychologists, and social workers).
- Focus groups can be used to identify (a) factors that motivate target providers to change, (b) how providers learn new practices (e.g., through instruction, written materials, or vignettes), and (c) the perceived barriers to adopting new practices.

ASSESSING COSTS AS THE BOTTOM LINE

The identification of organizational needs that warrant evidence-based behavioral health practices does not guarantee their implementation. Indeed, Bartels et al. (2002) note that, despite a growing database supporting interventions for common behavioral problems in late life, older adults are more likely than younger adults to receive inappropriate treatment. Barriers to the implementation of EBPs can occur at the philosophical, intellectual, or social organizational levels (Dickinson, Duffy, & Champion, 2004; Simpson, 2002). Thus, stakeholders might be wed to particular, incompatible models of mental health care; might have a lack of knowledge or skills; or might experience insufficient support (Corrigan, Steiner, McCracken, Blaser, & Barr, 2001). However, even when these hurdles have been successfully addressed, there remains one potential barrier to broadly implementing evidence-based practices: the bottom line. Regardless of efficacy or effectiveness, the question to be asked is, "Is there empirical support that the selected evidence-based practices can be implemented at a reasonable cost?" The answer falls into the realm of economic analysis.

A variety of economic evaluations—among them cost-benefit, cost-effectiveness, cost-utility, and cost-offset analyses—attempt to quantify the relative value of a given intervention to facilitate the decision process.

Cost-Benefit Analysis

To arrive at cost-benefit ratios, cost-benefit analyses calculate expenditures and health-related gains in common units, that is, condition-specific outcome measures. While cost-benefit analyses do not require the use of monetary units, they frequently resort to monetary units for convenience (Yates, 1994). For this purpose, researchers may attach a monetary value to survival or morbidity because they ask whether potential treatment gains warrant expenditures without considering other available treatment alternatives.

Cost-Effectiveness Analysis

Given the plethora of psychological and psychiatric interventions, today cost-effectiveness analyses are the most common form of evaluation found in the literature. In contrast to cost-benefit analyses, cost-effectiveness analyses compare a new intervention with an alternative. This type of economic evaluation assumes that health-care providers must choose between competing alternatives given limited resources, so that the decision to adopt one particular health-care strategy comes at the expense of forgoing another one ("opportunity costs"). Based on differences between interventions, the result of a cost-effectiveness analysis is relative and very sensitive to the choice of comparator alternatives. As pointed out in the "Primer on Cost-Effectiveness Analysis" (American College of Physicians, 2000), if an intervention is shown to be cost-effective, it does not necessarily save money (see also Azimi & Welch, 1998). "Cost-effectiveness" indicates a "reasonable cost" for an additional benefit, and cost-effectiveness analyses are used to quantify the relationship of greater effectiveness at greater expense compared with the status quo.

Concerned about the inconsistent methodologies applied to deriving the factors constituting the numerators and the denominators of the cost-effectiveness ratio, the Panel on Cost-Effectiveness in Health and Medicine convened in 1993 and recommended the following standards to facilitate the conduct and the consumption of cost-effectiveness analyses (Gold, McCoy, & Siegel, 1996). A cost-effectiveness analysis should specify:

- The perspective of the study, including funding sources, to identify potential bias.
- The gold standard as a cost-effectiveness analysis from the societal perspective.

- The societal perspective that considers all costs and benefits attributable to the intervention even if they do not directly involve the client.
- The characteristics of the sample with all inclusion and exclusion criteria.
- A replicable and generalizable costing protocol, including the original source of valuation for each item.
- Start-up costs (e.g., salaries, benefits, equipment costs, space, consulting and training costs).
- Operating expenses (e.g., direct costs such as labor, supplies, communication expenses; overhead such as administration and occupancy).
- Other direct costs (e.g., home care or nursing care, transportation expenses, home services), indirect costs related to loss of productivity (e.g., early retirement, sick leave due to follow up, side effects), and intangible costs related to quality of life (e.g., pain, suffering).
- The rationale for the comparator alternative, including a comparison of the frequency and intensity of the interventions.
- The use of the best currently available alternative to prevent artificial inflation of the ratio of differences in cost to differences in effectiveness.
- The window of time and the discount rate applied to costs and health effects to account for the effects of time on future dollars spent or accrued.
- The recommended time frame as the duration of the health state (e.g., meeting the diagnostic criteria for chronic depression) and that costs and health effects must be discounted at the same rate.
- A sensitivity analysis that considers the possible range of values for uncertain factors (e.g., costs, estimates of effectiveness, or discount rate). (A sensitivity analysis reports cost-effectiveness ratios based on fluctuation in those values and is especially important when the true effectiveness of a certain intervention with a particular population or in a particular setting is not known.)
- Detailed descriptions of the measures of clinical effectiveness.

Cost-Utility Analysis

In their 1996 report, the Panel on Cost-Effectiveness in Health and Medicine noted that clinical effectiveness may be measured in "dollars per case . . . averted, dollars per life saved, dollars per life year gained, and dollars per quality-adjusted life year (QALY) gained" (Gold, McCoy, & Siegel, 1996, p. 9). The latter measure distinguishes the specific term *cost-utility analysis* from the broader category of *cost-effectiveness analyses*.

QALYs acknowledge that the dichotomy of life and death does not suffice when quantifying the health outcomes of most interventions. Instead of coding "1" for "perfect health" and "0" for "death," QALYs adjust each remaining year of life for the estimated consequences of the health problems on overall wellness. The adjustment consists of multiplying the time alive by a numerical value called the "quality of life preference weight" for the health state at that time. QALYs, like other measures, still represent life years in units averaged across patients or clients, but the adjustment to the life years is thought to reflect the relevant quality of life changes.

Each cost-utility analysis must specify the procedure for arriving at the quality of life preference weights. Thus, it must provide details regarding the reliability and validity of the quality of life measures and stipulate whether people currently affected by a given health state or the general population completed the measures that generated the quality of life preference weights. Because the quality of life preference weights consider psychological and physical well-being, cost-utility analyses are frequently used to assess the outcome of psychological interventions. (For a critical review of the use of QALYs, see McGregor, 2003.)

Cost-Offset Analysis

Cost-offset analyses can be inherent in all the aforementioned forms of economical analyses. They involve a breakdown of all items for economic analyses into input and output costs (Yates, 2002). Input cost is the "total 'price' of all resources that make therapy possible, whereas output cost is the sum of all funds that other programs did not have to spend, because of the positive effects of therapy, plus all funds generated because of therapy" (Yates, 2002, p. 93). Given that modifiable behavioral risk factors have been reported to be the leading causes of mortality in recent years (Mokdad, Marks, Stroup, & Gerberding, 2004), cost-offset analyses most commonly examine the cost-saving effects of behavioral health-care measures on the utilization of medical services (for a review, see Cummings, O'Donohue, & Ferguson, 2002).

At first glance, these economic analyses may not seem of interest to practitioners who make decisions on the individual practitioner–patient level, because these analyses assess the effectiveness or utility of interventions at the societal scale. However, Ramsey and Sullivan (2002), recommend practitioners take an active role and allocate time to studying economic evidence for three reasons: (1) to have a voice in formulating national practice recommendations, which are typically affected by economic evidence; (2) to contribute through practitioners' detailed knowledge of individual applications to the literature on the effectiveness of particular interventions and subsequent utilization of other health-care-related services; and (3) to be able to advocate for the use of interventions that are cost-effective in the long-term, albeit at greater short-term expense. Moreover, reviews of cost-effectiveness analyses have consistently discovered methodological flaws and inconsistent reporting practices (e.g., Balas et al., 1998; Neumann, Stone, Chapman, Sandberg, & Bell, 2000) that have prompted some authors to suggest the typical peer review process be amended by the examination and verification of economic and clinical assumptions (Neumann et al., 2000). As Ramsey and Sullivan (2002) underscore, practitioners can and should participate in critically evaluating economic evidence for new interventions to improve the quality of published studies and to represent their interests and concerns.

Gordon Paul (2000) noted that practitioners and researchers have a common goal in trying to find sound and valid answers to the question, "What treatment, by whom, is most effective for this individual, with that specific problem, under which set of circumstances, and how does it come about?" (Paul, 1967, p. 44, cited in Paul, 2000, p. 4). Given the need for practitioners' representation in economic analyses, the call for cost-effectiveness analyses at the individual level has become louder (Bala & Zarkin, 2004; Fals-Stewart, Yates, & Klostermann, 2005; Yates, 2002; Yates & Taub, 2003), further dispelling the myths that EBP supports "cookie-cutter approaches" to treatment and a unidirectional relationship between research and practice (Addis, 2002; Addis, Wade, & Hatgis, 1999). Correspondingly, Strosahl (2002) recommends the development of cost-saving clinical decision pathways that facilitate the selection and incorporation of EBPs in different contexts. The workability of such pathways ultimately depends on practitioners' input. However, at this time, there are virtually no published data available on the economic feasibility of EBP in more naturalistic practice (versus academically affiliated, organized care) settings.

Studies that demonstrate successful implementation of EBP assume unconditional administrative support for training and maintenance (e.g., Schmidt & Taylor, 2002), including contingency management techniques that increase initial acceptability of and later adherence to EBPs (e.g., Andrzejewski, Kirby, Morral, & Iguchi, 2001). Accordingly, *training costs* are usually seen as one of the greatest concerns when implementing evidence-based treatments in clinical settings (Strosahl, 1998). This is especially true when training opportunities are not easily available, and indirect costs related to travel and loss of productivity (i.e., loss of client contact hours) increase. While the initial evaluation activities, such as the gap analyses or the needs assessment described earlier, may serve to justify the prospective expenses, additional funding is needed for start-up and maintenance costs.

As mentioned above, economic analyses assume limited resources: Adopting one practice also means forgoing another one that might be better suited for the particular context. Addis, Wade, and Hatgis (1999) list five questions that enter into the assessment of risk of adopting a given EBP:

1. Will the initial training and continued supervision suffice to guarantee best practice?
2. Will external constraints (such as session limits) decrease the effectiveness of the given EBP?
3. Will training provide the flexibility to modify the existing EBP while still capturing its process components, such that diverse groups of clients can be accommodated?
4. How will practitioners know when the EBP should be applied?
5. Will the client accept the EBP, or will the adoption of the EBP damage the practitioner's reputation or image?

MODIFYING AND IMPLEMENTING AN IDENTIFIED EBP

Modification of an EBP should be based on the underlying principles of the EBP and on detailed knowledge of the target problem. Any attempt at modification of an EBP by narrowly focusing on techniques rather than the underlying principles may result in removal or detrimental modifications to necessary critical components of the EBP.

When modifying treatments, Hayes and Follette (1992) indicated that the first important step is to identify potentially relevant characteristics of individual clients, their behavior, and the context in which the behavior occurs via an idiographic assessment. The collected data can then be analyzed in terms of the basic principles of the EBP. Any modification made must address the identified variables without omitting the underlying active ingredient.

Challenges to Expect in Implementing EBPs

Best practice in behavioral health care occurs when therapists, working in partnership with clients, rely on research evidence and their clinical knowledge and reasoning to implement effective interventions. Unfortunately several barriers exist that prevent the ideal model of EBP implementation, including structural, theoretical/principle, political, and client-based barriers.

Structural Barriers

Cranney, Warren, Barton, Gardner, and Walley (2001) identified structural factors as barriers that prevent practitioners from implementing EBPs. First, heavy workloads limit a practitioner's time and opportunities to learn EBPs, and further limit the opportunities for evaluating the effectiveness of a new EBP. Second, many practitioners simply do not read outcome literature (Cohen, Sargent, & Sechrest, 1986; Morrow-Bradley & Elliot, 1986; O'Donohue, Curtis, & Fisher, 1985), and therefore access to information about a new EBP can be difficult. Distinguishing among the myriad texts, journals, and training seminars can be overwhelming. Accessing the relevant resources has become easier with most journals offering online documents, but a practitioner would require several subscriptions to stay current with all new EBPs.

A common argument against EBPs is that they are an ivory-tower concept and not practical in real world (Gibbs & Gambrill, 2002). Methods of treatment delivery may not be practical or may have not been considered during treatment development. For instance, time constraints (number of sessions available) may make it impossible to follow the treatment as prescribed.

Theoretical/Principle-Based Barriers

It is not uncommon for practitioners to receive little or no training in methods that are supported by empirical evidence of efficacy. Graduate programs often provide extensive training in methods that are not supported by empirical research (Persons, 1995), and practitioners who receive training in non-EBP methods are being taught directly or indirectly that efficacy evidence is not important.

Practitioners may not have the knowledge or skills necessary to critically examine published research on EBPs. Skepticism of published research is commonly expressed by practitioners (Cranney, Warren, Barton, Gardner, & Walley, 2001). Further, clinicians may object to EBPs due to their lack of knowledge concerning processes, aims, and consequences. Practitioners have also reported that the dissimilarity between research samples and clinical samples limits the utility of empirically based treatments (Persons, 1995). The exclusion criteria employed in clinical trials can affect the generalizability of the findings if the research sample is significantly different from a clinical sample.

Practitioners may also object to utilizing an EBP if they feel that it ignores clinical expertise. EBPs that utilize a standardized protocol may not easily be adapted to clinicians' usual modes of treatment delivery (Persons, 1995). Gibbs and Gambrill (2002) note that many practitioners feel that EBPs with standardized protocols utilize a "cookbook approach" that may be perceived as ignoring client values and expectations. A significant challenge when implementing an EBP is using clinical expertise to integrate external research findings with idiosyncratic information regarding client characteristics and circumstances (Haynes, Devereaux, & Guyatt, 2002).

Political Barriers

EBPs may be perceived simply as cost-cutting tools, a way to save money and to promote revenues for the managed care industry (Gibbs and Gambrill, 2002). The notion that EBPs are simply a strategy employed by the managed care industry to increase profits is not based in fact. The majority of EBPs were developed by researchers who have no ties with the managed care industry. Furthermore, Straus and McAlister (2000) and Sackett, Richardson, Rosenberg, and Haynes (1997) noted that EBPs may increase, not decrease, cost.

Client-Based Barriers

Another concern about EBPs is that they ignore client values and preferences. Practitioners and clients may feel that an EBP ignores clients' values and expectations. Clients may feel they are forced to accept a one size fits all treatment that does not recognize them as individuals. Sackett et al. (1997) oppose this notion by pointing out that a hallmark of a good EBP is the consideration of client values and expectations. Additionally, studies have shown that the way in which an intervention is suggested to the client modifies the client's response (e.g., Hazlett-Stevens et al., 2002). Consequently, concerns about client acceptability might reflect a general unease regarding EBPs within the field, rather than challenges to their demonstrated economic and practical utility.

Addis (2002) noted that pharmaceutical companies successfully disseminated evidence-based interventions and concurrently generated a more active role for consumers in shaping clinical practice. In contrast, behavioral health consumers and their family members—specifically, geriatric populations, for whom visits to a behavioral health provider are associated with greater stigma—rarely demand the integration of evidence-based interventions into clinical practice. As a consequence, "important research findings often do not translate automatically into practice, while new and well-marketed products may sometimes achieve a greater market share than merited by their additional costs and benefits" (Mason et al., 2001, p. 2988).

Principle-Based Strategies

The level of training necessary for a practitioner to be effective depends on the level of clinical care that is needed by the client. Some clients may require in-depth and intensive treatment from a highly skilled practitioner, whereas others may be able to achieve treatment goals with minimal professional contact. Minimal professional interventions require only limited training for successful implementation. Therapies that rely on brief meetings, follow-up phone calls, or otherwise very little time from the therapist do not require the practitioner to fully understand the basic principles of treatment to be successful (Hayes, Barlow, & Nelson-Gray, 1999). However, EBP by professionals requires extensive preparation and time commitment for advanced level practitioners.

Hayes et al. (1999) describe practice guidelines as a product of the science-based practice. Practice guidelines are derived from the integration of basic science and theory and are evaluated on the basis of clinical replication of treatments. Scientists utilize basic research methods to test the underlying theories that are the foundation of effective treatments. Once the basic research on the underlying theories of a proposed treatment has been conducted, and researchers are satisfied with the outcomes, then treatment innovation may begin.

Treatment innovation rarely emerges from common sense; more often it emerges from the dynamic interplay between a detailed knowledge of the discipline and a detailed knowledge of the target problem (Hayes et al., 1999). Once a new treatment is designed, it is then evaluated based on single case designs, modified, reevaluated, placed through full-scale efficacy testing, and then disseminated to practitioners.

To fully understand the limits of the evidence of EBPs, a practitioner must be knowledgeable of the underlying theories and how the treatment components follow from the underlying theories. When attempting to apply the treatment within a new context or with a new population, it is imperative that the practitioner understands the underlying theories and can evaluate the extent to which the causal variables that affect the new context or population are addressed by the treatment.

Idiographic Assessment Strategies

Meehl (1954) used the term *clinical judgment* to refer to a method of aggregating data (informal, unstructured versus statistical, actuarial). Currently, clinical judgment more broadly denotes the judgments, inferences, observations, and practices of clinicians. The evolution of the definition of clinical judgment has lead to a widespread belief that empirical data have shown that the observations, thought processes, and beliefs of clinicians are seriously flawed (Westen & Weinberger, 2004).

The primary purpose of idiographic assessment is to collect information that increases the validity (i.e., the descriptive and prescriptive accuracy) of clinical judgments. The validity of clinical judgments will be strengthened to the degree that they are based on measures and strategies that are valid for the particular client, for the particular assessment context, and for the particular judgments to be made (Haynes & O'Brien, 1999). When faced with a new client, it is imperative that a clinician accurately identify the problem and any causal variables.

In the rare instance when a client presents with historical or current characteristics for which there is no research on treatment outcomes, group norms, or base rates, idiographic assessment is necessary to establish an accurate baseline in order to have valid comparisons of the treatment outcome. The idiographic assessment data would be the only information about the expected probability of the target problem. Without established group norms or without an idiographic assessment, a practitioner would not be able to accurately track treatment effectiveness.

To make valid predictions, a practitioner needs equivalent data from one case to the next. Without equivalent data the practitioner cannot make an accurate determination of causal variables. If variables included in each assessment were different for each case, then utilizing the assessment could not generate valid predictions (Westen & Weinberger, 2004). Further, not all research evidence on interventions is specific to an elderly population, or to contexts applicable to the elderly. The main issue is to determine whether a special treatment is needed for an elderly population or if the current treatment is adequate due to incorporation of the basic features of treatment that are specific to the elderly (Drake et al., 2001).

Clinical Utility

Once a treatment is deemed an EBP, it must be disseminated to practitioners in all areas of psychology. There are then three factors to be considered when determining the clinical utility of an EBP: feasibility, generalizability, and cost-effectiveness (Hayes, Barlow, & Nelson-Gray, 1999). A practitioner who wishes to modify an EBP should only modify it to improve on the three factors of clinical utility.

Feasibility refers to the extent to which an EBP can be delivered to patients in specific settings. The EBP can be modified in ways that it becomes more acceptable to clients (American Psychological Association, 1995). For instance, an EBP can be reduced in duration of each session or in the total number of sessions to increase client acceptability of the EBP. An EBP can also be modified to minimize any components of the EBP causing side effects or adverse reactions. *Generalizability* refers to the effectiveness of an EBP with many populations and a variety of practitioners, and in showing robustness of treatment effects (American Psychological Association, 1995). An EBP can be modified to allow a treatment designed for an adult population to be used with the elderly. Cohort effects must be brought into consideration whenever generalizing an EBP to an elderly population. When treating an elderly population, therapist factors such as age, gender, and race may affect clinical utility. Treatment robustness may not be as strong in real-world settings as compared to research settings. Thus, an EBP can be modified to allow for a different time frame for delivering treatment, or treatment may be interrupted to address extraneous variables that may affect treatment outcomes. Modifying an EBP to address *cost-effectiveness* can be achieved in a variety ways including length of sessions, total number of sessions, size of groups, and number of practitioners.

MAINTAINING AWARENESS OF NEW EBPs

Several strategies have been suggested for improving practitioners' access to current EBPs. In particular Proctor (2004) suggests that practitioners' ability to keep up with current EBPs may be enhanced through improved dissemination techniques, user-friendly writing styles, and changes in how service agencies evaluate and offer access to EBP.

The research community needs to improve and utilize greater "dissemination competence" (Huberman, 1994). Roos and Shapiro (1999) recommend condensed versions of research findings that clearly communicate results, with completely annotated and detailed reports. Furthermore, consensus statements regarding the generally agreed upon effectiveness of an EBP would be beneficial. Often individual studies state conclusions very differently from that of a systematic review of a body of studies. Lavis, Robertson, Woodside, McLeod, and Abelson (2003) suggest that consensus statements that convey clear ideas are more likely to have an influence on practitioners than discrete data.

Practice guidelines offer several advantages in enabling access to EBPs (Rosen & Proctor, 2003). Guidelines offer explicit instructions to practitioners, and practice guidelines based on several research studies can convey a clear idea about the underlying principles of the EBP. Manuals and guidelines need to be user-friendly, rather than steeped in academic jargon (Corrigan, Steiner, McCracken, Blaser, & Barr, 2001). Research reports must be explicit about the extent to which recommended EBPs have generally agreed upon evidentiary support (Proctor, 2004).

Service agencies can increase access to current EBPs through subscriptions to journals (both hard copy and online formats), newsletters, and Internet access to scholarly search engines. Face-to-face interchange between researchers and practitioners is also recommended (Proctor, 2004). Data on information dissemination suggests that interpersonal links are key to research use (Huberman, 1994; Innvaer, Vist, Trommaild, & Oxman, 2002). A final suggestion for the improving access to current EBPs is that agencies should establish research advisory committees or departments to collect, evaluate, and disseminate EBPs to practitioners.

REFERENCES

Addis, M. E. (2002). Methods for disseminating research products and increasing evidence-based practice: Promises, obstacles, and future directions. *Clinical Psychology: Science and Practice, 9,* 367–378.

Addis, M. E., Wade, W. A., & Hatgis, C. (1999). Barriers to dissemination of evidence-based practices: Addressing pracititioners' concerns about manual-based psychotherapies. *Clinical Psychology: Science and Practice, 6,* 430–441.

American college of Physicians (2000). Primer on cost-effectiveness analysis. *Effective Clinical Practice, 3*(5), 253–255. Retrieved from http://www.acponline.org/journals/ecp/sepoct00/primer.pdf.

American Psychological Association Task Force on Psychological Intervention Guidelines. (1995, February). *Template for developing guidelines: Interventions for mental disorders and psychosocial aspects of physical disorders.* Washington, DC: American Psychological Association.

Andrzejewski, M. E., Kirby, K. C., Morral, A. R., & Iguchi, M. Y. (2001). Technology transfer through performance management: The effects of graphical feedback and positive reinforcement on drug treatment counselors' behavior. *Drug and Alcohol Dependence, 6*(2), 179–186.

Azimi, N. A., & Welch, H. G. (1998). The effectiveness of cost-effectiveness analysis in containing costs. *Journal of General and Internal Medicine, 13,* 664–669.

Bala, M. V., & Zarkin, G. A. (2004). Pharmacogenomics and the evolution of healthcare: Is it time for cost-effectiveness analysis at the individual level? *PharmacoEconomics, 22*(8), 495–498.

Balas, E. A., Kretschmer, R. A., Gnann, W., West, D. A., Boren, S. A., Centor, R. M., et al. (1998). Interpreting cost analyses of clinical interventions. *Journal of the American Medical Association, 279*(1), 54–57.

Bartels, S. J., Dums, A. R., Oxman, T. E., Schneider, L. S., Areán, P. A., Alexopoulos, G. S., et al. (2002). Evidence-based practices in geriatric mental health care. *Psychiatric Services, 53,* 1419–1431.

Cohen, L. H., Sargent, M. M., & Sechrest, L. B. (1986). Use of psychotherapy research by professional psychologists. *American Psychologist, 41,* 198–206.

Corrigan, P. W., Steiner, L., McCracken, S. G., Blaser, B., & Barr, M. (2001). Strategies for disseminating evidence-based practices to staff who treat people with serious mental illness. *Psychiatric Services, 52,* 1598–1606.

Cranney, M., Warren, E., Barton, S., Gardner, K., & Walley, T. (2001). Why do GPs not implement evidence-based guidelines? A descriptive study. *Family Practice, 18*(4), 359–363.

Cummings, N. A., O'Donohue, W. T., & Ferguson, K. T. (Eds.). (2002). *The impact of medical cost offset on practice and research: Making it work for you.* Reno, NV: Context Press.

Dickinson, D., Duffy, A., & Champion, S. (2004). The process of implementing evidence-based practice—the curate's egg. *Journal of Psychiatric and Mental Health Nursing, 11,* 117–119.

Drake, R. E., Goldman, H. H., Leff, H. S., Lehman, A. F., Dixon, L., Mueser, K. T., et al. (2001). Implementing evidence-based practices in routine mental health services settings. *Psychiatric Services, 52*(2), 179–182.

Fals-Stewart, W., Yates, B. T., & Klostermann, K. (2005). Assessing the costs, benefits, cost-benefit ratio, and cost-effectiveness of marital and family treatments: Why we should and how we can. *Journal of Family Psychology, 19*(1), 28–39.

Gibbs, L., & Gambrill, E. (2002). Evidence-based practice: Counterarguments to objections. *Research on Social Work Practice, 12*(3), 452–476.

Gold, M. R., McCoy, K. I., & Siegel, J. E. (1996). *Cost-effectiveness in health and medicine: Project summary.* Washington, DC: U.S. Public Health Service, Office of Public Health and Science.

Goldman, H. H., Ganju, V., Drake, R. E., Gorman, P., Hogan, M., Hyde, P. S., et al. (2001). Policy implications for implementing evidence-based practices. *Psychiatric Services, 52*(12), 1591–1597.

Hayes, S. C., Barlow, D. H., & Nelson-Gray, R. O. (1999). *The scientist practitioner: Research and accountability in the age of managed care* (2nd ed.). Needham Heights, MA: Allyn & Bacon.

Hayes, S. C., & Follette, W. C. (1992). Can functional analysis provide a substitute for syndromal classification? *Behavioural Assessment, 14,* 345–365.

Haynes, R. B., Devereaux, P. J., & Guyatt, G. H. (2002). Editorial: Clinical expertise in the era of evidence-based medicine and patient choice. *ACP Journal Club,* March/April.

Haynes, S. N., & O'Brien, W. H. (1999). *Principles and practice of behavioral assessment.* New York: Kluwer Academic/Plenum Publishers.

Hazlett-Stevens, H., Craske, M. G., Roy-Byrne, P. P., Sherbourne, C. D., Stein, M. B., & Bystritsky, A. (2002). Predictors of willingness to consider medication and psychosocial treatment for panic disorder in primary care patients. *General Hospital Psychiatry, 24,* 316–321.

Huberman, M. (1994). Research utilization: The state of art. *Knowledge and Policy: The International Journal of Knowledge Transfer and Utilization, 7*(4), 13–33.

Ingersoll, G. L., Kirsch, J. C., Merk, S. E., & Lightfoot, J. (2000). Relationship of organizational culture and readiness for change to employee commitment to the organization. *The Journal of Nursing Administration, 30*(1), 11–20.

Innvaer, S., Vist, G., Trommaild, M., & Oxman, A. (2002). Health policy-makers' perceptions of their use of evidence: A systematic review. *Journal of Health Services Research Policy, 7*(4), 239–244.

Kaplan, R. M., & Groessl, E. J. (2002). Applications of cost-effectiveness methodologies in behavioral medicine. *Journal of Consulting and Clinical Psychology, 70*(3), 482–493.

Klein, K. J., & Sorra, J. S. (1996). The challenge of innovation implementation. *Academy of Management Review, 21*(4), 1055–1080.

Lavis, J. N., Robertson, D., Woodside, J. M., McLeod, C. B., & Abelson, J. (2003). How can research organizations more effectively transfer research knowledge to decision makers? *Milbank Quarterly, 81*(2), 221–248.

Mason, J., Freemantle, N., Nazareth, I., Eccles, M., Haines, A., & Drummond, M. (2001). When is it cost-effective to change the behavior of health professionals? *Journal of the American Medical Association, 286*(23), 2988–2992.

McGregor, M. (2003). Cost-utility analysis: Use QALYs only with great caution. *Journal of the Canadian Medical Association, 168*(4), 433–434.

Meehl, P. E. (1954). *Clinical vs. statistical prediction.* Minneapolis, MN: University of Minnesota Press.

Mokdad, A. H., Marks, J. S., Stroup, D. F., & Gerberding, J. L. (2000). Actual causes of death in the United States, 2000. *Journal of the American Medical Association, 291*(10), 1238–1245.

Morrow-Bradley, C., & Elliot, R. (1986). Utilization of psychotherapy research by practicing psychotherapists. *American Psychologist, 41,* 188–197.

Mueser, K. T., Torrey, W. C., Lynde, D., Singer, P., & Drake, R. E. (2003). Implementing evidence-based practices for people with severe mental illness. *Behavior Modification, 27*(3), 387–411.

Neumann, P. J., Stone, P. W., Chapman, R. H., Sandberg, E. A., & Bell, C. M. (2000). The quality of reporting in published cost-utility analyses, 1976–1997. *Annals of Internal Medicine, 132,* 964–972.

O'Donohue, W., Curtis, D. D., & Fisher, J. E. (1985). Use of research in the practice of community mental health: A case study. *Professional Psychology: Research and Practice, 16,* 710–718.

Oser, M., & O'Donohue, W. (in review). *Integrated care readiness assessment.*

Paul, G. L. (2000). Evidence-based practices in inpatient and residential facilities. *The Clinical Psychologist, 53*(3), 3–11.

Persons, J. B. (1995). Why practicing psychologists are slow to adopt empirically-validated treatments. In S. C. Hayes, V. M. Follette, R. M. Dawes & K. E. Grady (Eds.), *Scientific standards of psychological practice: Issues and recommendations* (pp. 141–157). Reno, NV: Context Press.

Poats, J., & Salvaneschi, M. (2003). Are you ready? *Health Care Technology.* Retrieved December 6, 2004, from http://www.hctproject.com/documents.asp?d_ID=1827.

Proctor, E. K. (2004). Leverage points for the implementation of evidence-based practice. *Brief Treatment and Crisis Intervention, 4*(3), 227–242.

Ramsey, S. D., & Sullivan, S. D. (2002). Weighing the economic evidence: Guidelines for critical assessment of cost-effectiveness analyses. In J. P. Geyman, R. A. Deyo & S. D. Ramsey (Eds.), *Evidence-based clinical practice: Concepts and approaches* (pp. 103–110). Boston: Butterworth-Heinemann.

Roos, N. P., & Shapiro, E. (1999). From research to policy: What have we learned? *Medical Care, 37,* JS291–JS305.

Rosen, A., & Proctor, E. K. (2003). *Developing practice guidelines for social work intervention: Issues, methods, and research agenda.* New York: Columbia University Press.

Sackett, D. L., Richardson, W. S., Rosenberg, W., & Haynes, R. B. (1997). *Evidence-based medicine: How to practice & teach EBM.* New York: Churchill Livingstone.

Schmidt, F., & Taylor, T. K. (2002). Putting empirically supported treatments into practice: Lessons learned in a children's mental health center. *Professional Psychology: Research and Practice, 33*(5), 483–489.

Simpson, D. D. (2002). A conceptual framework for transferring research to practice. *Journal of Substance Abuse Treatment, 22,* 171–182.

Snyder-Halpern, R. (2001). Indicators of organizational readiness for clinical information technology/systems innovation: A Delphi study. *International Journal of Medical Informatics, 63,* 179–204.

Stewart, T. A. (1994). Rate your readiness to change. *Fortune, 129*(3), 106–110.

Straus, S. E., & McAlister, D. C. (2000). Evidence-based medicine: A commentary on common criticisms. *Canadian Medical Journal, 163*(7), 837–841.

Strosahl, K. (1998). The dissemination of manual based psychotherapies in managed care: Promises, problems, and prospects. *Clinical Psychology: Science and Practice, 5,* 382–386.

Strosahl, K. (2002). Identifying and capitalizing on the economic benefits of primary behavioral health care. In N. A. Cummings, W. T. O'Donohue & K. T. Ferguson (Eds.), *The impact of medical cost offset on practice and research: Making it work for you* (pp. 57–89). Reno, NV: Context Press.

Westen, D., & Weinberger, J. (2004). When clinical description becomes statistical prediction. *American Psychologist, 59*(7), 595–613.

Yates, B. T. (1994). Toward the incorporation of costs, cost-effectiveness analysis, and cost-benefit analysis into clinical research. *Journal of Consulting and Clinical Psychology, 62*(4), 729–736.

Yates, B. T. (2002). Roles for psychological procedures, and psychological processes, in cost-offset research: Cost, procedure, process, outcome analysis. In N. A. Cummings, W. T. O'Donohue & K. T. Ferguson (Eds.), *The impact of medical cost offset on practice and research: Making it work for you* (pp. 91–113). Reno, NV: Context Press.

Yates, B. T., & Taub, J. (2003). Assessing the costs, benefits, cost-effectiveness, and cost-benefit of psychological assessment: We should, we can, and here's how. *Psychological Assessment, 15*(4), 478–495.

CHAPTER 3

Quality Management in Evidence-Based Service Programs

Hongtu Chen, Rodolfo Vega, JoAnn E. Kirchner,
James Maxwell, and Sue. E. Levkoff

Quality management (QM) is crucial to the success of the implementation of any evidence-based practice (EBP). After selecting and deciding on the appropriate EBP and redesigning the service system to meet the new EBP criteria, program developers have to ensure the quality of implementation so that the program can move toward its promised state of functioning. Just as the strategy for system redesign is to map out all the components necessary for the change, QM is the operational guarantee for the journey.

Quality management is a team approach that focuses on growth; growth is change from a coordinated approach and appropriately controlled pace, meeting commonly accepted standards and quality. Organizations without visionary leaders who are eager to find innovative paths often fail to make necessary changes. However, visionary leaders without QM skills also fail to help organizations grow.

Leadership is always crucial for making meaningful change. However, QM moves from a great-leader model to a system-control model. The great-leader model relies on a single person's good intention and willpower to make things happen. From an organizational point of view, having a "champion of change" is central to implementing any new plans or reorienting an organization in new directions. It is fortunate when an organization has a leader who not only sees the right direction but also leads people there. Any history textbook will testify to the validity of the great-leader model. However, the great-leader model is limited for several reasons: (1) a great leader is hard to find; (2) a great leader may not stay in one position forever, and departure of such a leader is often devastating to a program single-handedly initiated and cultivated by this person; and (3) a charismatic leader may be highly skilled at initiating projects, therefore creating so many projects that he or she cannot personally ensure their ongoing success.

Quality management moves beyond the great-leader model by developing a system that can operate on its own to ensure the quality of organizational development even when the leader or the original program initiator is no longer present. Originating from the industry and business world that emphasizes teamwork, collaboration, and analytic techniques, there are two basic approaches to quality management: the *administrative strategy* and the *evaluation strategy*. The administrative strategy, or people-based strategy, focuses on reorganizing and redirecting resources in individuals and organizations toward processes and outcomes devoted to quality improvement. The evaluation strategy, or data-based strategy, focuses on collecting and utilizing well-summarized information to monitor service processes and guide further decision making. In practice, both strategies can often be combined, but emphasis on one often depends on the availability of the skills of the people involved in a QM project.

ADMINISTRATIVE STRATEGIES FOR
QUALITY MANAGEMENT

The success of an EBP depends on the people working in a program. The administrative strategy for quality improvement requires a thorough understanding of people and their work. This people-based approach is particularly appropriate for EBP implementation, since an EBP in health care is primarily about helping, trusting, and improving people. Administrative strategies involve six steps: (1) building a team, (2) analyzing the work process, (3) determining quality indicators and standards, (4) gaining system support, (5) checking performance, and (6) problem solving.

Step 1: Building a Team

Building a Small Team

Structure is important for development and growth in quality management. The first structure is a small team (two to five people) of a core group who share similar key values and goals. The focus is on leadership building and developing opinion leaders, and the small group size will maximize collaboration to efficiency (e.g., decision making, meeting scheduling). The small team members are typically ahead of others in the organization in their thinking and understanding of the program to be developed, therefore may eventually influence others with their ideas and beliefs.

The first task of the small group is to reach a common understanding of the issue or project; common thinking and understanding will lead to unity, and unity will lead to organizational strength. All new projects need strength to proceed. In the QM context, a natural progression of consensus building can start with (a) sharing of common concerns (e.g., what if this whole project fails? what are potential dangers if we do not add extra effort in the current process?) and gradually move toward (b) reaching a general agreement about the necessity and importance of quality management and (c) discussing a general scope and action steps of the QM project.

The second task is to turn each of the core team members into an opinion leader who will influence other people in the organization. Therefore, the meetings should be organized in such a way that the participants feel free to express their opinions and feel respected for their ideas and contributions. The meeting organizer, who typically is the same person as the director of the EBP program, may sometimes feel pressure to make a trade-off between attaining common understanding and respecting individual opinion. A strategy recommended by negotiation and consensus-building experts is to identify a few things that can be agreed upon first, and then move on to encourage discussion while seeking new opportunity to identify another agreeable item. During discussion, the meeting organizer should build both a sense of group (i.e., "we as a group") and a clear respect of individual participants. Total respect leads to total participation; total participation leads to total commitment.

At the end of these meetings, the organizer can expect the participants to naturally energize others, or the organizer can give an assignment to each member to communicate with certain people and spread the message. It is sometimes the execution of this type of assignment that begins to turn a regular participant into a true opinion leader.

Building a Larger Team—the Quality Management Committee

A formal, larger team, designed to develop operational leaders, should gradually replace the informal smaller team. This larger team should be a new committee (which can be named Quality Management, Quality Control, or Quality Improvement Committee) operating separately from ongoing administrative or human resource department meetings. A separate structure will increase the status of a QM issue in an organization. More important, QM involves both organizational development (the agenda of the administration of an organization) and individual development (the agenda of the human resources department), and therefore its tasks usually cannot be subsumed by each of the existing departments.

The larger QM committee will typically face the following challenges:

1. Increasing and maintaining involvement of the whole organization.
2. Reaching common understanding of the mission of the project.
3. Analyzing and sharing knowledge of work flow and process.
4. Agreeing on and developing standards of quality.
5. Agreeing on strategies to execute the standards.
6. Agreeing on procedures for measuring and checking performance.
7. Reviewing results of performance measurement and identifying problems.
8. Developing and implementing solutions.

Involving People

The success of a QM effort depends on the extent to which the whole staff is involved in the project. If a change or project is merely perceived as a demand from a top leader or manager, true change in the behavior and attitudes of staff members is unlikely to follow. The first step in involving people and building a larger QM team is to recruit members for the QM committee who can represent all steps of the clinical flow. For instance, if the project is to implement an EBP that involves clinicians, nurses, direct service staff, administrative managers, human resources personnel, front desk staff, and case managers, then the QM committee should invite one person from each of these categories.

Full representation removes a typical problem of "them versus us"— that is, "they" (the managers or QM people) are checking on "us" (the staff, the workers). The "them versus us" division is a fundamental source of resentment and misunderstanding, which often leads to deception and covering up of quality flaws. Oftentimes, it is not laziness or reluctance to exert additional efforts, but the fear of being blamed or criticized that stops people from continuing a worthy cause. Among the many reasons that a team can fail (see Table 3.1), criticizing others and desiring self-importance are most detrimental.

The second step of involvement is a move from membership involvement to active involvement through expression and contribution. Since the purpose of the QM committee is to develop operational leaders, motivating and encouraging the committee members' participation is a key to improving their leadership quality. Active involvement is also an effective way to

TABLE 3.1   The Top 10 Ways to Guarantee Teams Will Fail in Your Organization

10. Don't listen to any new idea or recommendation from a team.

 9. Withhold from your teams any additional resources to help solve problems in their area.

 8. Treat all problems as signs of failure and treat all failures as a reason to disband teams and downgrade team members.

 7. Create a rigid system that requires lots of checks, reviews, and signatures to get permission for all changes, purchases, and new procedures.

 6. Get your security department involved in making it impossible for teams to get information about your business.

 5. Plant an "old line" manager on each team to keep an eye on everyone in your area.

 4. When you reorganize or change policies and procedures, never involve team members in the decision or even give them any advance warning.

 3. Cut out all team-member training.

 2. Lash out with your criticisms freely and withhold your praise and recognition.

 1. Above all, remember only you know best. Never let team members forget that.

Source: Adapted from Glenn M. Parker, *Personnel Journal, 73*(7), 69 (July 1994).

reduce or remove resistance, and recruitment for the QM committee should focus on representation rather than the likelihood that members will immediately reach consensus. The committee is not just a mechanism for reaching consensus but also a vehicle for learning and expression.

Building Consensus

Members of a larger committee will not agree with each other to the same degree as those in a smaller group, and therefore consensus needs to be built gradually. An experienced committee chair or facilitator:

- Knows the pace of consensus building and how much to accomplish during each meeting.
- Has general optimism toward the group process and resilience about frustration.
- Maintains clear goals revolving around the word "progress."
- Spends time building group identity and uses the accumulated "we-go' to supplement or replace "ego."
- Turns work into a fun and playful activity so that people will not be too defensive about their personal views.

- Studies participants' background ahead of time and is willing to learn and accept their concerns and resistance.
- Is comfortable guiding the group discussion and is able to stay neutral when it is necessary for the group process.
- Cares about the larger cause but also cares about each person's opinion and feelings.

A typical strategy for consensus building is the use of a voting process to reduce a list to a manageable size, but voting should not be the final or only step in the attainment of consensus. The spirit of consensus building should represent the very core of the democratic process: It encourages discussion to elicit the opinion of participating members and to gain insight; it allows everyone to have a chance to assent to the group's pursuit of an issue; it avoids a hasty decision or a decision dominated by a politically powerful voice. A typical consensus building session involves three major steps (set up, reduce alternatives, attain consensus), as outlined in Table 3.2.

Agreement on the importance and quality of the project should be the foundation and basic assumption of all QM works. Sometimes, asking an authority figure to support the opening session of the discussion about a particular project will create recognition of the importance of the project among committee members.

Disagreement that arises often has to do with concerns about practical benefits and costs, larger philosophical issues, or resentment caused by unfair treatment in the past. When a fundamental or major division is detected, either it needs to be addressed first or basic rules of engagement need to be

---

TABLE 3.2   Major Steps in Consensus Building

1. **Set Up**
   Write out the issue.
   Encourage group members to suggest many solutions.

2. **Reduce Alternatives**
   Reduce a long list (10+ items) by using a vote.
   Carefully discuss the remaining issues.
   Decide on evaluation criteria.
   Do a rating vote or a ranking vote.
   Identify areas of disagreement and discuss further.
   Vote again, if necessary.

3. **Attain Consensus**
   Discuss the outcome of the vote.
   Make sure everyone has been heard.
   Determine that everyone supports the decision.

set, before a group session continues. In general, disagreements are healthy and should be used to energize discussion; however, disagreement fueled by emotional baggage is a destructive force to any committee operation.

Managing Resistance

In a recent book, *Get Them on Your Side*, Samuel Bacharach (2005), director of Cornell University's Institute for Workplace Studies, identifies two crucial issues in the initial stage of change making in an organization: (1) securing legitimacy of the core agenda and (2) overcoming resistance. Securing legitimacy often requires the approval and support from senior managers, coalition building with peers, explanation of the Zeitgeist and trend of a particular time, or expertise and authority carried by the agenda initiators, who, in this case, are the small team of opinion leaders. When implementing an EBP program, the program initiators need to convince the senior leaders of the parent organization that quality improvement is a worthy move for the organization and why and how the evidence-based approach will benefit the organization.

Analyzing, managing, and overcoming resistance is important because stakeholders in the organization tend to have different agendas and concerns. Some resist the agenda or they resist those individuals who propose the agenda. In the case of an EBP implementation, there can be many individuals or groups resistant to the project. Boss A, for instance, is always concerned that policies maintain consistency with the tradition of the organization. Boss B resists every new proposal unless he is involved in the initial process and his opinion is accepted. The financial officer asks about the cost-effectiveness of the EBP program. The clinicians have doubts about how much the new EBP is better than their current practice. The secretary or office manager may not want to do anything extra. As the EBP implementer, it is important to identify and build allies, justify the approach, address concerns, and compromise as much as it is necessary.

Building an evidence-based mental health service for older adults often requires interagency or interorganizational collaboration, and people from different organizations may have different concerns and resistance toward a new project. For instance, in a *primary care clinic* where mental health professional seek opportunities for case identification and referral, the primary care providers' hesitation to get involved in a mental health project often has to do with their limited time and their competence in managing and treating mental health patients. A program developer should build components to address these issues, such as providing in-service training for primary care providers to improve their competence in handling or understanding patients, offering to review the charts of difficult cases, and making sure that the new procedure will not add more burden to the existing clinical flow.

In *aging services settings*, care managers are often concerned about the additional workload of a project, but also pleased with the possibility of getting help with some of their difficult cases. They would prefer a self-administered screening to a lengthy interview. In a *community-based mental health clinic*, even if the clinic leaders are willing to develop an evidence-based *geriatric* mental health service program, the mental health clinicians may hesitate to support such a program due to concerns about whether the new protocol will limit the number of sessions to the extent that it becomes incongruent with their regular practice or may even be linked to a possible financial loss. To gain the clinicians' support for implementing an EBP protocol, a certain level of flexibility should be built into the treatment protocol so that clinicians feel that they still maintain control in their everyday practice and decision making about the clinical process. Regardless of the setting, the resistance-free scenario is rare. Typically program implementers have to handle three groups of people with regard to their general attitude toward implementing a new clinical protocol: Those who are intrinsically interested should become allies; those who resist but require at least a response; and those who are in the middle need to be convinced of the merit of the proposed EBP.

Step 2: Analyzing the Work Process

A central component of QM is to understand and improve quality throughout the entire work process rather than just in key parts or at the end point only. However, the whole process is usually uneven in terms of having weak quality spots or potential quality issues; the areas requiring special efforts for improvement are usually countable, and improving them can significantly improve the quality of the whole process. An ideal QM effort needs to aim at both entirety and key points.

Two tools are typically recommended for analyzing the work process: the flowchart and the fishbone diagram.

Flowcharts

In quality improvement work, flowcharts are particularly useful for displaying how a process currently functions or could ideally function. A well-constructed flowchart can help the work team identify the necessary or redundant steps, define the boundaries of each step and identify responsibility, reveal problems or missing links, brainstorm solutions to a noticed problem, and develop a common knowledge base about a work process.

To construct an accurate and effective flowchart, the following six tips are recommended:

1. Clearly define each step in the process and describe the boundary with starting and ending points.
2. Complete the big picture before filling in the details.
3. Identify time lags and non-value-added steps.
4. Involve people who are directly involved in the work process.
5. Create a group work environment in which participants can be honest and accurately describe what really happens.

Fishbone Diagram

A fishbone diagram is also called cause-and-effect diagram or Ishikawa diagram because it was first developed by Kaoru Ishikawa of Tokyo University in 1943 for quality management in Kawasaki shipyards. The diagram has been widely used for planning, improving quality, and identifying problems and reasons (Ishikawa, 1982). The diagram is drawn to resemble the skeleton of a fish, with the main causal categories drawn as the bones attached to the spine of the fish (see Figure 3.1). The diagram assists teams in visually displaying the potential causes of problems or issues and in identifying root

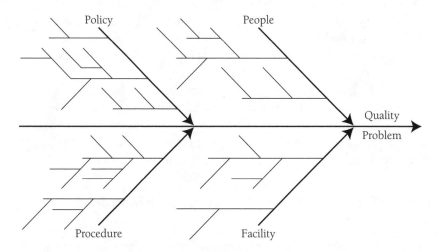

FIGURE 3.1   A fishbone diagram.

causes. One benefit of this method is that it helps to bring out a thorough exploration of the issues behind a problem.

The basic steps in constructing a fishbone diagram include the following:

1. Identify and list the problem/issue to be studied (e.g., how to improve the quality of the service through this program) in the head of the fish. Be sure everyone agrees on the problem statement before beginning.
2. Draw the fishbone structure with four (or five) categories of causes. The diagram usually arranges the causes into four main categories, while the contents and the number of these categories are not definite. In the health-service area, the categories of causes often include technical issues (facility), system issues (policies), logistic issues (procedure), and interpersonal issues (people).
3. Generate causes. An unstructured idea-generating technique (e.g., brainstorming) can be used to identify the factors within each category that may be affecting the problem/issue. The team should ask, "What are the procedural issues affecting the service quality of this program?" Repeat this procedure with each factor under the category to produce subfactors. Continue asking, "Why is this happening?" and put additional segments under each factor and subsequently under each subfactor. A structured brainstorming such as the 6-5-3 procedure (i.e., 6 people, 5 minutes, 3 ideas) is also helpful. Continue until there is no longer useful information obtained.
4. Analyze results. After team members agree that an adequate amount of detail has been provided under each major category, they should identify the "most likely causes" or "primary causes." The team should reach consensus on listing those items from the "most likely causes" category in priority order, with the first item being the most probable cause.

The main benefit of the fishbone diagram is to help users organize their thoughts and structure the quality improvement process. Use of the fishbone diagram is most successful when the work group is succinct, seeks the truth, remains open to different ideas, pursues each line of causality back to its root cause, and considers splitting up overcrowded branches.

Step 3: Determining Quality Indicators and Standards

The third step is to reach a common agreement on the indicators and standards of quality for the quality improvement process. The group should select and define quality in a measurable way for each major step of the service process.

In recent years, federal resources have been used to develop quality indicators in the health-care field (e.g., APA Task Force on Quality Indicators, 1999). Definitions and references for quality indicators that can be used to measure the quality of mental health care (e.g., Table 3.3) are readily available. Therefore a committee often needs to decide which indicators to choose and focus on. For those who start new QM work in a particular area, a stepwise approach is recommended of starting with one indicator at each service step, and adding another indicator only when the use of the previously proposed indicator is grasped by both the QM committee and the frontline service staff.

Although deciding on a quality indicator is relatively easy, it takes weeks and months for the service staff to truly integrate such a standard and for the standard to become an organizing force in their daily work. It is important to fully involve frontline service staff in the decision process regarding the choice of an indicator as they are most likely to be significantly impacted by the change.

Once a quality indicator is selected, a natural next step is to decide on the expectation or standard corresponding to the indicator. For instance, if the group agrees that "% of people receiving screening among the clinic visitors" will be an indicator, the committee can then decide on standards, for

TABLE 3.3 Typical Quality Indicators Used in Mental Health Services for Elderly People

- Regular use of standardized instruments, clinical examination or other methods (e.g., Geriatric Depression Scale) to screen older adults at risk for depressive disorders.

- Percentage of older adult clients in a given health plan receiving psychiatric evaluations whose records indicate explicit evidence of assessment, by history or formal measure, of current or past mental health problems or substance use disorders.

- Percentage of older adult clients with depressive disorder or dysthymia in a given health plan who receive specialized services from a provider with appropriate training and expertise.

- Percentage of patients in a given health plan with a diagnosis of depressive disorder who have received psychotherapy in a given year.

- Percentage of patients in a given health plan with new-onset cognitive impairment who receive a medical workup that includes a sequence of evaluative tests until a positive finding indicates a potential cause of new-onset cognitive impairment.

- Percentage of patients in a given health plan with major depressive disorder, moderate or severe, receiving an appropriate dose of antidepressant medication.

- Number of panic attacks in a given time interval compared to a pretreatment interval.

example, 50% of all of the visitors to the clinic who are 60 years of age and above be screened by the end of the first month of the project. Depending on manpower, clinic operations, and screening procedures, 50% might not be a low standard for the beginning month. Setting an appropriate standard is critical because if the standard is set too high, the staff will feel discouraged and possibly angry about the unrealistic QM work; conversely, if the standard is set too low, staff members may lose their respect for and consequently ignore the QM work. It might be wise to set a range, with the highest standard on one end, and the lowest tolerable standard on the other end. Sometimes, an agency will receive information about national standards or standards described in a nationally recognized protocol. A typical strategy is for the agency to use the national standard as the lower bar and to set up its own standard as a higher bar. An agency can decide to use not only higher but also more criteria than the minimum requirements of a national standard.

A standard is a tool to guide behavior, not to suffocate individuals' creative solutions to a local problem. After a standard is determined and agreed upon, argument about the standard could be healthy for both staff involvement and organizational development. The argument about standards often arises during the time of quality checking. For instance, a quality evaluator who checks the implementation of a new program that integrates mental health service with primary care may feel dissatisfied with the degree of communication between the mental health clinicians and primary care providers. The quality indicator written in the protocol states, "There should be evidence that mental health clinicians used the patient medical records that can be shared by primary care providers." The quality evaluator finds no evidence. The director of the integrated service program has to explain that the mental health clinicians decided not to use the common medical record as a means for communication because (a) primary care providers do not like to read the lengthy and detailed notes typically made by the mental health clinicians and (b) both primary care providers and mental health clinicians share the same office and they find face-to-face communication about a mental health case to be more effective. As a result, they decide to change the originally suggested method of communication and practice what they believe to be more effective for communication. The evaluator investigates the situation and helps the team write a new *indicator of communication*, which states, "Mental health clinicians make a note of initiating a conversation with the primary care provider about the mental health case, and share further diagnostic and treatment information with primary care provider if requested."

Analysis of the relevance of a quality indicator is a complicated science. For the frontline service men and women, it is often impractical to expect the decision regarding the choice of a quality indicator to be based on whether there is evidence of the short-term and long-term benefits as well as side effects. A thoughtful and reasonable discussion among all parties is always the best approach for assessing the indicator; if this approach fails, an external or internal authority on the subject matter can be invited to settle the disagreement and identify a solution. Sometimes, another standard may need to be added or an additional period of time needs to be allowed for further observations.

Step 4: Gaining System Support

Once a standard range for the quality indicator is set and agreed upon, the lowest bar becomes a driving force for the immediate work, and the highest bar becomes a long-term aim. To ensure the successful execution of the project, the QM committee may want to propose a financial incentive plan to the organization's management team. A more politically effective way is to have an administrative manager or the financial officer as a regular member of the QM committee and ask that member to help develop an incentive plan to submit to the leaders of the organization on behalf of the QM committee.

Quality management success often requires support from both the department of human resources (HR) and department of administration (AD). The HR department is able to integrate quality-related performance into the existing incentive system. A monetary incentive (bonus) can be used to improve performance of an entire group, and promotion can be used to reward the exceptional or accumulated contribution of an individual. The collaboration between the QM committee and the HR representative involves the development of an algorithm to assign the weight for each performance indicator in order to calculate the distribution of the whole bonus.

The AD is in charge of how leaders or managers are selected in each group, and how the reporting system is arranged to ensure progress and timely identification of problems. The collaboration between QM and the AD focuses on increasing the status of the quality issue on the high-priority list and helping AD develop concrete action steps to reflect such a priority adjustment.

While working on the system toward improving quality, the QM committee should recognize that in the earlier phase of a new practice, especially when developing a mental health service for older adults with challenging situations, quality indicators may not be the best way to check the progress and promise of a program. A period of watchful waiting should be allowed before formal evaluation of the program. For those programs serving ethnic minority populations, exploration and time for making and correcting mistakes might be the best pathway toward finding a culturally specific way to improve and maintain high quality services.

In the initial period of developing the EBP, the QM committee should also aim to support the new practice by finding ways to stabilize the performance of the practice (before checking on qualities). There are generally two approaches to stabilizing the performance of an EBP: (1) For those who choose to follow a well-established evidence-based practice guideline, the approach involves helping the whole practice team become familiar with the guideline. Some project leaders post the key quality points or performance indicators on a bulletin board or in a place easily accessible to the team members, while others arrange group discussions to help team members quickly grasp the major points of a protocol. The most successful learning method involves making small-step progress, reviewing progress regularly, rephrasing key points, and forming study partnerships. (2) For those who develop a new EBP when there is no appropriate EBP guideline available for a specific service situation, a number of measures can be employed to help stabilize the performance, including the development of a practice manual to operationalize the procedure and protocol. One approach is forming a fast-track support system in which the problems reported by the frontline service staff will be immediately discussed together with the QM members or leaders, and a solution will be generated. When a service staff member realizes that his or her report of a problem receives the highest priority and a quick supportive response, it sends a clear signal about the importance of both the work and the worker. Awareness of importance is the key to conscious action toward quality work.

Step 5: Checking Performance

Checking the performance against quality standards is an imperative step for the success of QM in the real world. It is the QM committee's duty to identify methods for checking performance such as (a) specialty checking, (b) checking on each other, (c) self-checking, and (d) checking fidelity.

Specialty Checking

Checking by someone specialized in quality assessment can be very effective when the person who is checking has expertise in the subject matter. A person external to the organization may generate more respect, but an internal person may see and hear more that is crucial for further improvement. The specialty checking can be counterproductive when an "us versus them" division occurs between the working team and the checking person. Therefore, an amiable and nonthreatening person is a better choice for performing specialty checking than a serious and authoritative figure.

Checking on Each Other

Checking on each other works well at the initial implementation phase as it helps familiarize team members with the quality standards and how one's work relates to the standards. The method works best when the coupling team members are similar in terms of age or background, or when a trust relationship has already been developed. The method can be beneficial if it is combined with other checking methods, such as specialty checking.

Self-Checking

Self-checking is the cornerstone of all quality management. Self-checking is a method that every employee uses on a regular basis to systematically assess the quality of his or her own work. For instance, the QM committee can help a project team develop a checklist that each worker can use for self-reflection at the end of each day's work. Some checklists may simply include the specific content or checkpoints of the work, while others may use a more generic style to focus on unsolved problems and opportunity for improvement. If the group members decide that the self-checking card not be shared with others, this method should be combined with other methods to ensure the standard used by each individual is congruent with those of others.

The QM committee can help improve the success of the implementation of the identified checking method by, for instance, associating people's name or ID next to each major checkpoint. A successful arrangement of accountability is helpful for giving credit to those who deserve it and identifying who should be responsible for mistakes and errors. However, overemphasis on individual-based accountability can be detrimental to the team spirit, especially during the initial phase of setting up a new project.

Checking Fidelity

Assessing whether an intervention or service is appropriate (i.e., its benefits exceeding risks by a wide enough margin) and whether care adheres to professional standards are two basic measurement approaches in the quality of care literature (IOM, 2001; Wells et al., 1993; Brook, Chassin, & Fink, 1986;

Donabedian, 1980). In implementing an EBP, practitioners often face the challenge of fidelity issues. Fidelity is the degree to which the program is implemented as the original EBP model or principle and assumes (a) the original EBP model is one of high quality; (b) the implemented program is of high fidelity if it resembles the original EBP model; and (c) programs that faithfully implement original EBP models have better outcomes. However, when EBPs move from the research environment to the real world where contextual variables play an important role in determining whether a reputed EBP model should be modified or not, it becomes more difficult to exactly replicate an original EBP.

Regardless of whether fidelity refers to an EBP *model* fidelity, *principle* fidelity, or *component* fidelity (see in Chapter 2 on modifying an EBP), the tool or the scale used to measure fidelity should include concrete indications that the key elements of an EBP model or principle have been implemented as intended. Many established EBP programs (e.g., assertive community treatment, integrated treatment for dual disorders, family psychoeducation) have developed detailed fidelity scales that can be used to check fidelity from the beginning to the mature stage of the program (Bond et al., 2000). Again, if there is any conscious change or adaptation made to the original model during the implementation, the fidelity tool may also need to be modified. Fidelity assessment is most valuable when the implemented program is intended to faithfully replicate an established EBP model.

Step 6: Problem Solving

This final step, problem solving, is of central importance in QM. All previous steps focus on building quality while this step is about improving and fine-tuning quality. A well-established model for fine-tuning the quality improvement process is the Plan-Do-Check-Act (PDCA) cycle. The PDCA cycle was originally conceived by Walter Shewhart, a pioneering statistician who developed process control in the Bell Laboratories in the United States during the 1930s. It was later adopted from the 1950s on by the QM authority, W. Edwards Deming (1986). Recently, the Institute for Healthcare Improvement has promoted the use of this tool as a way to improve quality in health services. The model provides a framework for the improvement of a process or system.

The PDCA cycle emphasizes that an improvement program must start with careful planning, must result in effective action, and must move on again to careful planning in a continuous cycle. Once a problem is identified, or its status reviewed and analyzed, in the *planning* stage, the beauty of the PDCA cycle is its arrangement for testing the solution first in the *do* stage, and depending on the results of the testing in the *check* stage, the solution will be further adopted in a larger scale or abandoned in the *act* stage. The fine-tuning of the service process lies in the ability to identify and solve particular quality problems through (a) problem analysis and (b) solution analysis.

Problem Analysis

The identification of a quality problem is only the beginning of understanding the problem. Team members should give serious thought and discussion to investigating the problem, including the severity and impact of the problem as well as the and likelihood that the problem can be corrected. The trend of the problem and the underlying causes of the problem also require consideration. If the trend indicates that the problem is a temporary matter or it is already in the process of being corrected, watchful waiting is the appropriate response. More formal analysis should be undertaken if signals indicate that the problem is not disappearing. The causes of the problem may be easily found by reviewing the process flowchart. Conducting problem analysis may also be the time to modify the process flowchart. For any given problem, there can be a large number of multiple causes. The causal analysis should stop at the level where the identified causes are likely to be corrected.

Solutions Analyses

Identifying effective, evidence-based, and affordable solutions is the key to the success of all QM efforts. In an attempt to systematically seek solutions and develop a coordinated action plan, the QM committee may encounter a number of issues.

   Long-term versus short-term solutions. Oftentimes, the QM committee feels that it is facing a trade-off between a long-term solution that will address the root of the problem and a short-term solution that requires fewer resources and time. For instance, the committee may come to a conclusion that changes must be made at the human resources department level (e.g., the agency's policy regarding recruitment of employees, incentive procedure, and staff promotion need to be further changed). But it is never easy to actualize high-resource solutions in an organization, especially when suggestions come from a small committee. Sometimes, one has to take a strategic position to immediately execute that which *can be done* and gradually work on those that *should be done*. It is also possible that the QM committee and the administrative leaders can work out an experimental solution (e.g., developing an incentive method only for staff involved in the particular program) without involving any agencywide changes.

Solution versus execution. The concept and importance of execution (i.e., implementation) has been increasingly recognized in business and management fields. However, our understanding of the gap between having an EBP protocol and its implementation, between identifying a solution and executing it, does not mean that we can easily reduce the gap. When a solution does not work out as expected, the QM organizers should at least determine whether the problem is in the plan or is due to the imperfect implementation or execution of a good idea or plan. One execution issue that often hinders all work progress is inefficiency in supervision. Previous work on improving health service quality has found that supervision is one of the main determining factors of success of QM, and that good supervision is well organized, encompasses a variety of methods, and has a style healthy for problem solving and work planning (PHC MAP, 1993). Table 3.4 lists some typical questions for assessment of supervision activities.

Problem-based coping versus anxiety-based coping. An unsolved problem often creates anxiety in an administrator's mind. At the moment of high anxiety, some people are able to refocus on the problem and rationally search for solutions, while others would like to find anything that can reduce the anxiety experienced. For example, a mental health program focusing on referring identified elderly people with depression to a mental health clinician continually has low participation rates. The program leader is puzzled. While agonizing on finding solutions at a QM meeting, one person mentions that her cousin who is a professor in health services research may be willing to come to give a talk as training for the program staff. The leader quickly approves the training idea and feels relieved of the uncomfortable feeling of not being able to find a solution. Inviting a speaker may not cost much, but time can be costly: two to six months can easily pass in scheduling the talk, waiting for the speaker, receiving training, and finally realizing that the training has little effect on solving the real problems. Those administrators who realize their frequent use of anxiety-based coping may benefit from participating in a training workshop that focuses on improving problem-solving skills or emotional management.

Using Tools

Since so many people have difficulty analyzing problems and finding solutions, some computerized tools can assist in these tasks, in addition to

TABLE 3.4   Self-Assessment of the Quality of Supervisory Activities

- Do supervisees meet with their supervisor at least once a month?
- Does the supervisor have regular staff meetings?
- When scheduled supervisory activities are cancelled, are they rescheduled?
- Do supervisors use the following methods during supervision?
  —Observation of end products (e.g., service delivery, counseling session)?
  —Asking supervisees about what problems they have been having?
  —Team approach to problem identification and solution?
  —Review of records, supplies, or conditions of facility?
  —Assessment of outcomes or other evaluation data?
- Are supervisees given adequate support through the supervisory system?
- Do supervisors make comments aimed at improving service quality?
- Do supervisors allow the supervisee adequate time to talk about problems?
- Do supervisors establish a good rapport with the supervisee?
- Do supervisors praise good performance?
- Do supervisors help their supervisees:
  —organize and plan their work?
  —identify problems?
  —make recommendations, respond, or take action on the problems or issues raised by the supervisee?
- Do supervisees feel free to discuss problems with the supervisor?
- Are supervisory activities, including problems identified and follow-up activities, recorded?

the traditional pencil and paper tools such as the fishbone diagram. Concept mapping and idea processing are increasingly popular. Concept mapping is a way to discover knowledge, and organize and represent ideas in a picture or diagram. First developed by Professor Joseph D. Novak (1990) of Cornell University, concept mapping allows quality administrators to use what they already know about a particular problem and develop new knowledge through the expansion, extension, or observed relations among the known facts. It is particularly suitable for quality control teamwork since it encourages input from various participants in a structured fashion. One of the premiere resources on concept mapping is the Web page developed by Dr. William Trochim at http://www.socialresearchmethods.net/mapping/mapping.htm that offers links to countless resources. Specifically, concept mapping involves the creation of diagrams consisting of nodes or cells each containing a concept or idea. One particular tool for concept mapping, and also for creative writing and quality management, is the Axon

Idea Processor, developed by Dr. Chan Bok from Singapore (http://web. singnet.com.sg/~axon2000/). The program provides a sketchpad for users to visualize and organize ideas. When ideas are shown as graphical objects and their relationships shown as links, the user can maintain the big picture at all times. Details can be hidden from view or retrieved from the background. Those who have used this program find it helpful for many purposes including solving a research problem. The idea behind Axon products is "to provide an environment that supports thinking." These tools in general can be very attractive and helpful, but like many other management tools, they require the participants to have healthy organizational learning skills.

EVALUATION STRATEGIES FOR QUALITY MANAGEMENT

Evidence-based practices are established through a combination of rigorous empirical research and the body of knowledge accumulated from clinical experience. In practice, however, the EBP is often implemented with a population and in a setting vastly different from the one in which it was validated. How can we ensure that the selected EBP has been implemented in a manner that conforms to the way in which the EBP was originally developed and implemented? What are the tools and criteria required to adapt the EBP to the client or tailor the EBP to the setting?

Evaluation is a systematic way of collecting information to monitor the quality of an EBP implementation. The EBP approach assumes that there is a model, based on well-established evidence, that will improve quality of service at a particular setting. Evaluation, however, assumes that the reputed EBP model may not work as well as promised in the new context. Standing between the ideal and the reality, evaluation tries to find the story about the difference (Dowie, 1998).

The administrative strategy, or the people-based strategy, if operating well, can be quite effective in ensuring and improving the quality of services. In contrast, the evaluation strategy, or the data-based QM strategy, does more to inform about than ensure the quality of work. Both administrative and evaluation strategies involve evaluative effort, but the administrative strategy of QM primarily relies on intuitive judgment and perception or sporadic indicators, whereas evaluation strategies are based on carefully designed methods and systematic data collection. The four main steps of evaluation are (1) identifying evaluators, (2) evaluation planning, (3) process evaluation, and (4) outcome evaluation.

Step 1: Identifying Evaluators

Most program administrators find it critical to have a professional evaluator on board to help assess the program. Typically, a service program developed in a community-based clinical setting may need only a part-time professional. Therefore, an EBP program developer can either hire an internal evaluator and share the evaluator with other programs under the same parent organization, or employ an external evaluator as a consultant. One disadvantage of an external evaluator is that the evaluator is remote from the program development. Nevertheless, with the availability of telecommunication tools, it is becoming a common practice for a consulting firm to send out well-trained program evaluators to help evaluate programs across several states. A good source for looking for such consulting firms is a Web page (www.eval.org/consultants.htm) provided by the American Evaluation Association.

In an ideal situation, an evaluator will work intimately with program developers not only by monitoring the progression of a program, but also by providing relatively unbiased perspectives and feedback to program developers. In a slightly less ideal situation, an evaluator will perform a perfect evaluation and write an impressive report but rarely communicate with program developers. A commonly unfortunate scenario is when the evaluator is waiting for the program developers for guidance on next steps while the program developers are waiting for the evaluator to tell them what to do next.

Step 2: Evaluation Planning

The initial meetings between program developers and the evaluator should address the logic of evaluation and the administration of the evaluation.

Logic of Evaluation

A good evaluation plan must be logical, making sense to all parties regardless of whether they have met. Initial meetings between the evaluator and program planner should focus on the purpose of the evaluation effort, defining data collection and use of data, the audience for the evaluation report, and what will be learned from the program. Program goals will impact the evaluation process. For instance, a program developer may simply want to develop a service that can help people in the community, or he or she may want to share information about a new and creative program. One way to organize an evaluation plan is to sort issues by questions. In the case of implementing an EBP for older adults, the following questions can be asked:

- About providers: What is the evidence that the provider behavior has been changed?
- About consumers: How many older adults have been served by this program? How much have their conditions/situations improved after receiving the service from this program?
- About program implementation: Did the original EBP work as a clinical protocol? What was adapted? What was altered? What is the main innovation? What is the scientific basis for all the decisions and actions?

After addressing these initial questions, developing a logic model will help one move from a general evaluation discussion to a more detailed conceptual frame before heading toward designing methods and procedures.

Logic Model

A logic model is a diagrammatic representation of a theoretical framework that describes the logical linkages among program resources, conditions, strategies, short-term outcomes, and long-term impact. A logic model is a useful tool employed by program evaluators and program planners as a guide to the implementation of an intervention and evaluation plan (Julian, 1997). A well-designed logic model can assist in clarifying the approach to, and possibly ensuring the quality of, the adaptation of an EBP by helping program stakeholders understand and reach common agreement regarding which specific components of the EBP to include and their potential outcomes.

Although there are no specific guidelines or standard format for creating a logic model, its components should include the answers to the basic core questions (i.e., who, what, when, where, how) regarding the EBP intervention and the expected short-term and long-term outcomes of the program. The answers to those questions yield a description of the context in which the EBP will be implemented so that the practitioners can compare the similarities and differences between the context of origin and the context of implementation.

Based on the logic model, the evaluator can develop a design and data collection plan. The administrator should review the design and its associated administrative issues. Some of these design issues include feasibility of the proposed plan (e.g., Is this design doable, given the time and resource limit?), data source (e.g., Where will the data come from? What is the sampling strategy?), data type (e.g., Quantitative or qualitative data? What is the best method for answering the evaluation question?), measures and tool selection (e.g., What scales and indexes will be included? Are they linguistically and culturally sensitive to the serviced population?), and data use and analysis plan (e.g., How will the data be processed and analyzed?).

Administration of Evaluation

Typically, the program developer, evaluator, clinical managers, and staff members need to work together to solve administrative and logistical issues relevant to the evaluation, such as: (a) how to manage the evaluator (e.g., What is the cost estimate for hiring the evaluator? How often should they meet? To whom should the evaluator report?); (b) data collection logistics (e.g., Is the equipment used to collect the data available? Is there space for collecting confidential data? Can the interruption to the clinical flow be reduced to a minimum?); (c) cultural considerations (e.g., Are the methods, tools, and people selected for collecting data culturally appropriate?); and (d) Institutional Review Board (IRB) issues (e.g., Where to get IRB approval for this evaluation project? How will the evaluator help with the IRB application?).

Step 3: Process Evaluation

Process evaluation is designed to describe and analyze how a program is conceptualized, planned, and implemented. It is used to (a) determine whether the program is implemented as planned, (b) provide feedback to program developers so that the intervention can be adjusted and enhanced, and (c) reveal strengths and weaknesses of a program. Process evaluation addresses the central question of an EBP implementation: What happened in the implementation process? A well-performed process evaluation will clarify the process of the steps in the implementation of an EBP, thus providing insight about effective or problematic steps or components.

Many process evaluations do not particularly improve an EBP program. There are two general types of process evaluations. One is the *descriptive process evaluation* that aims at an exhaustive description of the program by including many variables regarding when, where, what, and how the service is delivered. In the end, a book of descriptive data is often beyond a community health center's analytical capacity. Table 3.5 lists some typical questions of a simple descriptive process evaluation.

To make a process evaluation more directly useful for the EBP program developers, one can also perform a *heuristic process evaluation* with an emphasis on both asking questions relevant to the key concerns in implementing an EBP in the real world and on learning from the answers. Table 3.6

TABLE 3.5   A Sample of Descriptive Process Evaluation Questions

- Why was the program introduced into the community or organization?
- What is the program? What are the components?
- What kind of principles or guidelines is this program based on?
- What changes or adaptations have been made to the original guideline?
- What is the composition of the program team?
- How effective is staff?
- How are they trained?
- What are roles and responsibilities of staff?
- How satisfied are staff with the program?
- How are clients recruited?
- How often is the program population being contacted?
- What design changes may be necessary to replicate the program elsewhere?
- What are the program costs? Have there been changes in funding? What about future funding?

presents some sample questions from a heuristic process evaluation. Almost all of these questions have no fixed answers. For instance, readiness is considered as one of the barriers or enablers standing between an EBP model well supported by scientific evidence and the successful implementation of such a model in the real world. On the one hand, there is never full readiness in any organization. On the other hand, motivational readiness (e.g., enthusiasm) may compensate for low knowledge readiness. Although readiness is a complicated issue, program developers may at a certain point want to know where the team and the organization was before the program started, and the best way to obtain this information is to document or assess it through a thoughtful process evaluation.

The EBP implementation field is rich in its contextual variability, thus providing ample sources of knowledge development. To truly understand what makes an EBP program work, one can seldom be assured by reading a research article or from listening to an expert. Self-guided learning is crucial in finding the most appropriate way to develop a program that fits the local cultural, service, and organizational settings. A heuristic process evaluation is a tool for learning about the key issues in the process of program implementation, though it may not be a tool for determining the best approach to improving a situation. Process evaluation is a tool for collecting the relevant information that may help reflective program developers to find their answers on their own.

TABLE 3.6   Ten Questions for a Heuristic Process Evaluation of an Evidence-Based Program

1. Was there an assessment or discussion about the organizational and staff readiness prior to the implementation of the EBP program? Was there effort to improve the readiness?

2. Is there an EBP guideline or protocol that has been the basis of this EBP program? If not, are there any evidence-based principles to guide this EBP effort, and how did you find or come up with these principles?

3. Was the original guideline or principle altered in the current practice, and what is the rationale for the choice of adaptation?

4. Which part of the original guideline or principle was adhered to in the implementation? What is the method to monitor and measure model fidelity?

5. What is the mechanism or method (e.g., team meetings, financial incentive, training) to ensure the progression and quality of the implementation of the EBP program?

6. Is there a systematic effort to document aspects of the new practice (e.g., where, when, who, what)?

7. Is there evidence that, as a result of the EBP project, changes or improvements in practice (e.g., practitioner's behavior, service procedure) occurred?

8. Is there an organized effort to evaluate the outcome or the impact of the EBP program?

9. Is there a method in place to collect comments and suggestions for the program? What are the main complaints or comments about this program from staff members? What are the main complaints or comments about this program from the users of this service program?

10. What are the major barriers to the EBP implementation? What are the solutions that work well, or things that make it successful? What are the problems that are still unresolved?

Step 4: Outcome Evaluation

Outcome evaluation addresses the ultimate question about an EBP program: Does it work? Does it make any differences, as intended? What improved as a result of this program? Since outcome evaluation is about testing a causal–effect relation, the best outcome evaluation has to be conducted via a well-controlled, double-blind, randomized trial. For most community-based program developers, resources usually will not permit the luxury of conducting a randomized trial. Therefore, what can typically be achieved as an outcome evaluation is a confirmatory examination about the impact of a program.

The most important aspect of an outcome evaluation is clarity about the logic of the outcome evaluation for the program (Wholey, Hatry, &

Newcome, 1994). There are several clear logical loops in every outcome evaluation:

- Outcome evaluation attempts to find evidence for a normally simple causal–effect relationship before the program starts, during the program intervention, and after experiencing the program.
- Outcome evaluation activities can be organized based on three simple steps: define data, collect data, and use data.
- Each step can be summarized under three themes: who, how, and what (see Table 3.7).

Outcome is only one of the possible quality indicators of a developing service program, and to what degrees this particular quality indicator is correlated with other quality indicators is often an empirical question. In other words, one could have carefully designed and implemented a program (i.e., good planning and implementation) and find poor outcomes; or one may follow exactly the same protocol as a well-recognized EBP protocol (i.e., high fidelity) and not find as good an outcome as expected. When no significant outcome is found, it does not necessarily mean that the program has no

TABLE 3.7   Basic Structure of Outcome Evaluation for a Service Program

Step 1: Define data

   Who are the target clients?

   How is the service delivered?

   What outcome changes do we expect to see?

   —What time frame (short-term, intermediate, long-term)?

   —What aspect of changes (participation, knowledge, and attitude changes, satisfaction, clinical symptoms)?

   —What other variables need to track and control?

Step 2: Collect data

   Who will collect the data (and who is going to pay for the cost)?

   How to collect data (i.e., develop instruments, such as questionnaires, interviews, surveys, document review)?

   What are the data sources (e.g., current program records and data collection, new data source)?

Step 3: Use data

   Who will analyze the data? Who will read the report?

   How to analyze the data?

   What kind of report needs to be written?

impact at all. Sometimes it only means that the selected outcome measures were not valid or not sensitive enough. The effect of an EBP program may not show immediately in its clients; significant impact can happen at an organizational level (e.g., staff behavior, staff interests, organizational interests) and tremendously improve an organization's readiness for the next trial of a new program.

When a positive outcome is found, caution needs to be taken in interpreting the finding that suggests the success of an EBP, despite the urge for promoting the program. Given the methodological constraints (e.g., not using a randomized control trial) usually found at a community health center and given the possibility of multiple causes and variables, positive outcomes may not indicate a causal–effect relationship at all, or may only indicate a partial causal relationship. Sometime, a positive finding may simply result from the Hawthorn effect—that the participants are aware of being observed and therefore perform unusually well. Finally, the QM attitude is probably the best approach to an outcome finding: In QM, evaluation is only a strategy to collect information for further attempts to improve the quality of practice.

DISCUSSION

The purpose of EBP is to improve the quality of care. The principles of quality improvement or quality management (QM), with its focus on learning and managing continuous improvement efforts, are congruent with the general orientation of EBP.

Learning addresses the known and unknown. Quality management requires cumulative learning about processes of working and methods for improving. Similarly, EBP encourages reliance on existing knowledge and evidence (the known) in empirically based clinical decision making. For an EBP implementer who is always conscious of the gap (the unknown) between established knowledge and actual practice settings, EBP implementation becomes inseparable from an evaluative effort to continuously monitor the progress and outcomes and to capture the information necessary for justifying modification and innovation.

Management establishes productive orders and reduces counterproductive chaos. The people-based administrative strategies of QM are attempts to build up quality-conscious orders in people's minds, routines, and problem-solving styles, and to reduce the chances for repeated oversight and mistakes. The data-based evaluation strategies of QM are attempts to establish accurate information about the status and outcomes of the implemented

EBP program while reducing the chaos contributed by inaccurate expectation, assumption, denial, and other subjective bias. Both the administrative and evaluation strategies of quality improvement are two complementary and inseparable methods to ensure the success of EBP implementation.

What remains most challenging to the success of implementing EBPs is probably beyond the scope of the standard QM doctrines. The contextual factors, such as cultural resistance of consumers toward mental health care, lack of organizational support or incentive to foster changes, and unfavorable changes in the financial environment of larger systems continue to be the source of many persistent barriers and complexities, presenting challenges to EBP programs.

REFERENCES

APA Task Force on Quality Indicators. (1999). *Final Report*. Retrieved from http://www.psych.org/psych_pract/tf_toc.cfm?pf=y.

Bacharach, S. (2005). *Get them on your side*. Woodbury, NY: Platinum Press.

Bond, G., Williams, J., Evans, L., Salyers, M., Kim, H. W., Sharpe, H., et al. (2000). *Psychiatric Rehabilitation Fidelity Toolkit*. Human Service and Research Institute. Retrieved from http://www.tecathsri.org/product_description.asp?pid=10.

Brook, R. H., Chassin, M. R., & Fink, A. (1986). A method for detailed assessment of the appropriateness of medical technologies. *International Journal of Technology Assessment in Health Care, 2*, 53–63.

Deming, W. E. (1986). *Out of crisis*. Boston: The MIT Press.

Donabedian, A. (1980). *Explorations in quality assessment and monitoring: Vol. 1. The definition of quality and approaches to its assessment*. Ann Arbor, MI: Health Administration Press.

Dowie, R. (1998). A review of research in the United Kingdom to evaluate the implementation of clinical guidelines in general practice. *Family Practice, 15*(5), 462–470.

Institute of Medicine (IOM). (2001). *Crossing the quality chasm: A new health system for the 21st century*. Washington, DC: National Academy Press.

Ishikawa, K. (1982). *Guide to quality control*. Asian Productivity Organization.

Julian, D. A. (1997). Utilization of the logic model as a system level planning and evaluation device. *Evaluation and Planning, 20*(3), 251–257.

Novak, J. D. (1990). Concept maps and Vee diagrams: Two metacognitive tools for science and mathematics education. *Instructional Science, 19*, 29–52.

Parker, G. M. (1994). The top 10 ways to guarantee teams will fail in your organization. *Personnel Journal, 73*(7), 69.

The Primary Health Care Management Advancement Programme (PHC MAP) Series of Modules, Guides and Reference Materials. (1993). Aga Khan Foundation.

Wells, K. B., Rogers, W. H., Davis, L. M., Kahn, K., Norquist, G., Keeler, E., et al. (1993). Quality of care for hospitalized depressed elderly patients before and after implementation of the Medicare prospective payment system. *American Journal of Psychiatry, 150*(12), 1799–1805.

Wholey, J. S., Hatry, H. P., & Newcome, K. E. (Eds.). (1994). *Handbook of practical program evaluation.* San Francisco: Jossey-Bass.

CHAPTER 4

Culturally Grounding
Evidence-Based Practice

Ramón Valle, Elizabeth Stadick, Jane Latané, Virginia Cappeller,
Monica de La Cerda, and Gregory Archer

THE CONCEPTUAL BASE

Introduction to Culturally-Grounded Evidence-Based Practice

Culture matters. It is a central filter for sending, receiving, and interpreting communications. It is the medium for generating interactions among individuals, groups, and organizational systems. It is the backdrop for evaluating which ideas and actions are compatible with our own. Moreover, cultures provide both explicit and implicit sets of rules to guide their members, with most of the rules being implicit.

Culture matters because it plays a key, but often unnoticed, role in everyday mental and behavioral health practice (Chen, Kramer, Chen, & Chung, 2005; Beiser, 2003; Tseng & Strelzer, 2001; Rogler, Malgady, Costantino, & Blumenthal, 1987). Practitioners constantly deal with different cultures when working with different populations. Whether young or old, whether ethnically diverse or ethnically mainstream, clients and consumers of behavioral and mental health services bring culture to the practitioner–consumer interaction table. Practitioners do the same, as they come from many different organizational, professional, and personal cultures. The idea of culture permeating all forms of human relationships likewise extends to the evidence-based practice (EBP) field (Ruiz, 2004, Williams, 2004). If we look at the EBP movement closely, we see that it brings its own distinct cultural stamp to the encounter between practitioner and client. For example, the EBP field makes use of specific terminology; it has rules regarding the implementation of practices; and it has its set of core values, centering on the empirical validation of the practice methods and measures. Best practices, coming from professional consensus, are acceptable, but practices that have been tested for efficacy or effectiveness are preferable. The standards are high, but understandably so, especially where consumer interests are concerned.

Unfortunately, however, when it comes to making cultural considerations an explicit part of behavioral and mental health interventions, both the behavioral and mental health fields are less explicit, as is the EBP arena (Bernal & Sharrón-del-Río, 2001; Brach & Fraser, 2000). A corrective step can be taken by building on the strength of the EBP movement, namely, its avowed purpose to assure that the most effective, soundly tested, and objectively verified intervention methods and measures are used on identified needs or problems (Gerrish & Clayton, 2004; Areán et al., 2003; *Evidence-Based Practices*, 2003; Bartels et al., 2002; Goldman, Thelander, & Cleas-Goran, 2000; Chambless et al., 1998). A thorough examination of cultural inputs into the planned interventions will be clearly in sync with EBP values (Ruiz, 2004; Pinn, 2003; Brach & Fraser, 2000; "Guidelines," 1993). In the project described in this chapter, the Positive Aging Resource Center, Targeted Capacity Expansion (PARC TCE) program and its Partner Sites (Tiempo de Oro in Phoenix and the Health Improvement Program for the Elderly in Tucson) faced the challenge of bringing culturally grounded evidence-based practice (CG EBP) to mental and behavioral health interventions with elderly patients in multicultural environments (Chen, Kramer, Chen, & Chung, 2005; *Review*, 2004; Lambert, Donahue, Mitchell, & Strauss, 2003; Montoro-Rodriguez, Kosloski, & Montgomery, 2003; Guarnaccia, Martinez, & Acosta, 2002; Lau & Gallagher-Thompson, 2002; Levkoff & Sanchez, 2003; Li, McCardle, Clark, Kinsella, & Berch, 2001; Levkoff, Levy, & Weitzman, 2000).

Designing and Implementing the Culturally Grounded EBP Framework: The Conceptual Underpinnings

Culturally grounded evidence-based practices require clear design elements and working principles (Valle, 1998). In this section we discuss five working principles critical to CG EBP: (1) accounting for between-group heterogeneity; (2) accounting for within-group differences; (3) designing organizational cultural inputs on parallel tracks; (4) generating a sound CG EBP theory base; and (5) separating client situational factors from cultural considerations.

Principle 1: Accounting for Between-Group Heterogeneity

CG EBP begins with a clear recognition of *between* group differences relative to the populations that are to be included in the planned intervention. The CG EBP practitioner understands that one size does not fit all in community-based mental and behavioral health intervention efforts. In a multicultural society such as the United States, cultures can live next to each other, with many points of contact and accommodation. However, they do not always mesh in terms of their language, custom, and philosophy about health care, especially where mental health concerns are present. In its cognitive–behaviorally based intervention, the Health Improvement for the Elderly Program, targeted an ethnically mixed, Jewish, Euro Anglo, and Latino/Hispanic clientele residing in the greater Tucson metropolitan area, along with the mostly Euro ethnic, but rural population in the Marana Valley. In its prevention-intervention program, Tiempo de Oro targeted two Latino/Hispanic groups in the El Mirage and Guadalupe communities in the Greater Phoenix area, with Guadalupe also including a Pascua Yaqui elderly population. Tiempo de Oro also implemented the program with another primarily Latino/Hispanic comparison group in the Hamilton community, likewise within the Greater Phoenix area. Additionally, Tiempo de Oro included other ethnic populations residing within its target catchments. It was evident that both Partner Sites consciously addressed between group variations throughout all of their program implementation stages.

Principle 2: Accounting for Within-Group Differences

The CG EBP model also starts with an expectation of *within* group heterogeneity. Not all members of any specific group, whether ethnically or demographically defined, think and act alike. Acculturation is always at work. Intragroup variation must be understood, and group stereotypes avoided regardless of the fact that the intervention may focus on a specific ethnic or generational group. At the point of their respective proposal submissions, the two PARC Partner Sites clearly reflected the recognition of this principle within their respective programs. Tiempo de Oro planned to work in three Latino/Hispanic communities, which also included other resident ethnic groups. From the onset Tiempo de Oro identified the need to modify its community outreach strategy to reflect the norms operating in each of the target communities. The Health Improvement Program for the Elderly likewise recognized the need to accommodate the expectations of its rural (Marana and urban Tucson) Euro ethnic (Jewish and Anglo) as well as Latino/Hispanic program participants. For example, the Health Improvement Program for the Elderly was aware from the start that not all the Jewish clients would have had a direct familial experience with the Holocaust; that not all the Anglos came from the same backgrounds; and that the Hispanics ranged from traditionally oriented monolinguals through bilinguals, to more acculturated English speakers only.

Principle 3: Designing Organizational Cultural Inputs on Parallel Tracks

The CG EBP effort has to operate simultaneously along four parallel tracks. First, one component of the effort requires the preparatory work of defining and describing the diverse target population(s) while paying close attention to the demographic, cultural, and regional characteristics of the target population(s). Second, this defining and describing activity has to continue through all of the project implementation phases. Third, the CG EBP effort has to closely consider the cultural content of the intervention programs and how the content will be monitored and documented. This is especially necessary because everyday cultural activity is very subtle, and presents itself as background, rather than surface content. This content is often best picked up through qualitative methods in which the important details and nuances of cultural exchanges within the immediacy of practitioner–client interactions can be recorded. PARC and the Partner Sites found it helpful, as suggested by the Substance Abuse and Mental Health Services Administration (SAMHSA), to preplan the quantitative and qualitative data collection (McDonel, English, & Brown, 2003; Borson, Bartels, Colenda, Gottleib, & Meyers, 2001). The Partner Sites maintained a variety of qualitative data collection and documentation procedures to accompany the specific quantitative outcome measures that were used. For example, for qualitative data collection, the Partner Sites employed such techniques as maintaining outreach activity logs, incorporating some open-ended interview and participant response questionnaire items, and keeping case notes to capture those observations that might be made in phone conversations and in staff exchanges. Fourth, it is important to ensure that the instruments and protocols are both language and age appropriate. One noteworthy innovation was the design and implementation of a Web-based data collection system used by the Health Improvement Program for the Elderly, which had been designed by the University of Arizona Center on Aging evaluation team. It enabled each treatment site to easily enter data immediately from their remote locations in the field, and allowed the program leadership to view all site records for ongoing quality control purposes. This system was a useful tool, making the quantitative data readily available for analysis.

Principle 4: Generating a Sound CG EBP Theory Base

As strongly recommended in the literature (Miranda, Nakamura, & Bernal, 2003; Miranda, Azocar, Organista, Muñoz, & Lieberman, 1996), practitioners need a cohesive conceptual base from which to operate. One potential problem is that there are many varied definitions for the term *culture*. The search for working approaches yielded two compatible frameworks within which to couch the idea of culture. First, Dilworth-Anderson and Gibson, (2002, p. S56) provide a viable working definition: "Culture is a set of shared symbols, beliefs and customs that [helps] shape individual and/or group behavior." Second, using this springboard, PARC and its Partner Sites also turned to a complementary formulation whereby the intended CG EBP could be clustered around three key areas of human interaction: (1) the language and communication processes of the target group; (2) the relational ties within different groups; and (3) the group's underlying values and belief systems (Valle, 1998, 1988–89).

1. The *language and communication processes* of the target group. For this project, the idea of language was broadened to incorporate all aspects of cultural and cross-cultural communications, including nonverbal exchanges, an understanding of the principal holidays observed by the target client group, and the art or artifacts preferred and used by the group members. Even seemingly small matters, such as how different client groups preferred to address themselves became important considerations. For example, the Tiempo de Oro project leadership and the prevention specialists working in the town of Guadalupe realized right away that the correct way to identify the Pascua Yaqui group was to always use that formal designation. The term "Yaqui" by itself is insulting arising from the Anglo and American Indian conflicts of the 19th and 20th centuries. PARC and its Partner Sites recognized that language and communication processes were the cornerstone of their CG EBP interventions, as this is the most common place where the practitioner and the participant exchange actual understandings around intended messages. The Partner Sites therefore prepared accordingly. They did so not only by hiring language-compatible personnel but also by preparing their informational materials to match the communicational styles of their target populations.

2. The *relational ties* within different groups. Regardless of whether the culture is of ethnic, regional, or generational origin, understanding the manner in which relational ties are formed and maintained is crucial to CG EBP. Equally important are the *expectations* of the parties involved as to how these relationships play out over time. Additionally, the practitioner must remain attentive to how relationships are established and maintained within different social environments, for example, relationships in the home, workplace, or the clinic. PARC and the Partner Sites recognized that the practitioners would be coming with specific interventive orientations and targets: CBT therapy on the part of the Health Improvement Program for the Elderly, and mental and behavioral health

prevention–intervention focused home visits, community education session, and prevention support group workshops on the part of Tiempo de Oro. Additionally, Tiempo de Oro recognized that each of the communities of Guadalupe, El Mirage, and Hamilton had their own social structures, cultural broker, and gatekeeper paths of entry (Florio & Raschko, 1998; Valle, 1998–89), as well guidelines as to how social relationships were to be maintained over time. The Health Improvement Program was alert to the same concerns with regard to its own very different Jewish, Anglo, and Latino/Hispanic groups, as well as rural versus metropolitan elderly clientele.

3. The group's underlying *values and belief systems*. Practitioners must understand and operate within all the different subtleties of the client's underlying values and belief systems, while recognizing that they will bring their own organizational and professional and personal values into the planned interventions. Values are ever-present in the situation where a CG EBP takes place. Both Tiempo de Oro and the Health Improvement Program for the Elderly maintained ongoing staff training to continuously heighten the knowledge and skills of their practitioners in recognizing the subtleties in the world views and outlooks of the different client and participant populations.

Figure 4.1 summarizes the different sets of cultural orientations that come into play within any given CG EBP practice engagement. It also highlights why PARC and its Partner Sites immediately recognized that they would need to follow a coherent set of cultural principles if they were to make evidence-based sense of their varied interventions in the multicultural working environments. As noted, practitioners bring their own cultural orientations expectations and those from their sponsoring organization (Gutterman & Miller, 1989), as well as those from the EBP field (Miranda et al., 2005), into the practice encounter. Consumers likewise carry their own ethnic group, age cohort, regional, and local influences, along with their individual worldviews and normative expectations. In a CG EBP context, all have a bearing on the practice that is being empirically experienced and documented.

Principle 5: Separating Client Situational Factors from Cultural Considerations

Beyond the notion of culture itself, the CG EBP practitioner must differentiate situational factors from cultural variables. Mixing situational and cultural factors together can lead to confusion both at the practical level of implementing the interventions and in the data analysis. In this project,

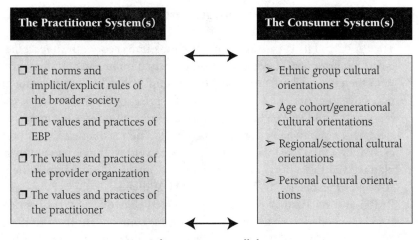

FIGURE 4.1   The multicultural context of CG EBP.

PARC and the Partner Sites developed five guiding principles for maintaining awareness of situational factors:

1. PARC and the Partner Sites recognized that apart from cultural considerations, *health literacy* presents particular problems for the successful implementation of mental and behavioral health interventions as well as health interventions in general (Health Literacy, 1999). For example, the target group members may not have received basic health and mental health information, or informational materials might be geared toward too high a grade level, even when translated into the participants' primary language. Partner Sites realized that plain-language content, both spoken and written, would be needed if their proposed interventions were to take hold and be subsequently appropriately measured.
2. The PARC–Partner Sites also recognized that their CG EBP practitioners would need to be aware of *low literacy or illiteracy* (Kaestel, Campbell, Finn, Johnson, & Mikulecky, 2001). Basic illiteracy (i.e., the inability to read and write) is distinct from health literacy (i.e., the inability to understand the health or mental health information that is provided).
3. The PARC group understood that the *underlying issue of nonparticipation* in the planned intervention, might not be culturally based. Rather PARC and the Partner Sites prepared their CG EBP practitioners to assess for the presence of comorbid conditions, which could block active

participation or bring about irregular participation. Comorbid factors can pose major impediments to even the best planned CB EBP effort.

4. The PARC and its Partner Sites likewise took into account the *impact that a person's prior history* could have on participation in and continuing on with the proposed interventions. For example, the client or participant may have experienced a chronic lack of service availability and accessibility and could still be holding on to remembered prior discriminatory treatment (Marawha & Livingston, 2002). The residual effects of perceived, or actual, past discrimination might very well interfere with the planned CG EBP effort—apart from any normative cultural impediment (*Unequal Treatment,* 2002; Whaley, 2003; Williams, 2003).

5. PARC and its Partner Sites also concurred that their CG EBP practitioners needed to be aware that *low income* status by itself, apart from cultural considerations, can interfere with addressing mental and behavioral health concerns. The circumstances of participants with extremely limited incomes could create barriers, particularly around ineligibility for services.

The CG EBP interventions used in this project were not by themselves sufficient to overcome all of the barriers and problems just described. For example, the PARC Partner Site efforts could not change the income or literacy levels of their clients. Moreover, as Tiempo de Oro experienced, they could often not find the appropriate Spanish language health resources to handle all of the comorbidities of their low income Hispanic and Pascua Yaqui program participants. The Health Improvement Program for the Elderly leaders and field staff could not change the residual effects of past discrimination that some of their clients had experienced (e.g., that some of their Jewish clientele had been directly seared by the Holocaust).

Additionally, it was observed that, when working in the cultural arena, the PARC TCE and its Partner Sites experienced a truism in that in CG EBP practice, everything comes wrapped together. Cultural and situational factors are intermingled and layered. Latinos were not just monolingual Spanish speakers, nor were they all poor. Some of the Jewish elderly communities were Holocaust survivors, some were family members of survivors, and some lived in the United States their entire lives. It is the culturally attuned practitioner's role to use the proposed CG EBP model as a guide to sort out what does and does not fit into the understanding of culture, as well as what does and does not fit into social status considerations.

In practice PARC and its Partner Sites found that they could keep both the cultural and situational factors apart within the designs of their respective programs, and, moreover, that they could account for the differences in

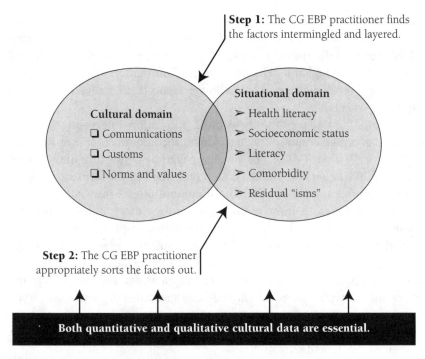

Step 1: The CG EBP practitioner finds the factors intermingled and layered.

Cultural domain
❏ Communications
❏ Customs
❏ Norms and values

Situational domain
➤ Health literacy
➤ Socioeconomic status
➤ Literacy
➤ Comorbidity
➤ Residual "isms"

Step 2: The CG EBP practitioner appropriately sorts the factors out.

Both quantitative and qualitative cultural data are essential.

FIGURE 4.2   The CG EBP model in operation.

both their quantitative and qualitative analyses. Figure 4.2 summarizes the sorting processes involved in applying the CG EBP model.

PROGRAM EXPERIENCES AND OUTCOMES: APPLYING THE CG EBP FRAMEWORK

The intent of this discussion is to provide illustrations of the application of some, but not all, of the principles described in the preceding section. For maximum effectiveness, a CG EBP must be supported through documentation processes that include both quantitative and qualitative data gathering activity.

Applying the CG EPP Model: A Qualitative Look at Engaging the Community

Tiempo de Oro was funded to conduct a behavioral health prevention intervention using a three-tiered strategy, namely, (1) *presentations* and community education events (e.g., health education lecture/discussions);

(2) *workshops* in the context of discussion-oriented support groups, each extending over a specified number of sessions (usually four to six), within a leader-guided discussion format; and, (3) *home visits* focused on providing pertinent mental and behavioral health information to less ambulatory community residents (e.g. those who were enrolled or eligible to receive meals-on-wheels).

Tiempo de Oro's culturally attuned prevention–intervention strategy followed accepted community engagement techniques (Florio & Raschko, 1998; *ElderVention*, 1997). The process began by contacting the key gate-keepers of the target communities. A second step was the formation of community advisory councils in each of the communities, before launching any part of the threefold intervention: prevention–intervention workshops, community educational events, and home visits. These first two steps extended over the first nine months of the project, and the return for the consistent outreach work was gatekeeper buy-in regarding the intervention and subsequent successful enrollment of participants into the prevention–intervention trial. Moreover, Tiempo de Oro succeeded in the eventual transformation of its community advisory groups into stakeholder constituencies (Gittell & Vidal, 1998) who continue to see themselves as an integral component of the overall effort.

CASE 4.1: REACHING OUT TO AND ENGAGING ETHNICALLY DIVERSE COMMUNITIES IN A CG EBP CONTEXT

During the second annual PARC TCE meeting held in Phoenix in March, 2004 (which included all of the nine SAMHSA-funded demonstration projects, the SAMHSA project officers, and PARC faculty), a strong contingent of members of Tiempo de Oro's (TdO) community advisory councils from both towns actively participated in the meetings. The community advisory council members came early, stayed late, and collaborated with all of the professionals to offer both sound advice as well as their appreciation for TdO's behavioral and *mental health prevention services* that were now coming into their respective communities. They sat through, at times, technically oriented discussions, sharing their insights using both local Spanish and English terminology. As Elizabeth Stadick, the TdO coordinator told the PARC TCE attendees: "This level of participation did not just happen."

Beginning in the fall of 2002, TdO targeted two primarily Latino/ Hispanic communities in the greater Phoenix area—the towns of El Mirage and Guadalupe—with the intent of bringing its three-tiered behavioral and mental health prevention services to the underserved ethnically diverse elderly residing there. It took 9 months of ongoing input to obtain approval to launch the intervention, and another 9 months of steady recruitment for a total of 18 months of concerted outreach effort by TdO in both communities before the prevention intervention took hold in both target communities. However, after these 18 months, not only were the community education events, the prevention–intervention workshops, and the home visits solidly in place, but the members of both community advisory councils were also asking to be trained as mental health aides. And, they were at the Second Annual PARC TCE meeting broadening their advising roles.

As Elizabeth Stadick described to the PARC TCE attendees, TdO had a defined outreach plan that involved (1) having an intimate grasp of the demographics of the two communities before they even got there; (2) investing time in actively listening to, and appropriately waiting for answers from their key community contacts (i.e., its gatekeepers and cultural brokers); and (3) tailoring and adjusting their approaches to the local community (e.g., taking into consideration language issues, outlooks, and expectations). For example, the TdO project leadership recognized early on that, despite the fact that both El Mirage and Guadalupe are largely Spanish-speaking Mexican American communities, they are distinctly different with different indigenous organizational structures. El Mirage resembles a 1950s community. Its elderly, many of whom had been migrant farm workers, are the community gatekeepers. Guadalupe, in contrast, resembles a Mexican town, with a church and plaza at its center. This community was settled in the late 19th and early 20th centuries by native Pasqua Yaqui peoples, followed by a number of Mexican families whose leadership role continues to the present. The Pasqua Yaqui Indian subgroup, while speaking Spanish, nonetheless maintains a strong tribal-elder decision-making system. An example is that TdO had to first ask permission of the Guadalupe Pascua Yaqui tribal leadership before any pictures of their elderly could be used on TdO brochures.

In her presentation at the meeting, Elizabeth noted, "If there is a lesson from the TdO effort to implement the mental health prevention-education program, it's that there's a lot of waiting before moving ahead." This waiting meant no knocking on doors to recruit workshop participants, and no holding of group or individual educational and home visit counseling sessions until the community advisory councils of both communities gave their permission. This waiting likewise involved attending many community events and meetings, and being willing to have one's patience tested by the community gatekeepers until permission to enter was received. It also meant being willing to report to SAMHSA month after month that there were still no clients in the program because the community relations contacts and procedures needed to be in place first.

In assessing the community connection process, it is evident that several CG EBP principles were applied. First, the Tiempo de Oro Partner Site went into the field with (a) a clear awareness of its own organizational culture; (b) a recognition of the different cultures and decisional structures of the two target communities and their varied normative orientations; (c) an expectation that language differences would be encountered; and (d) while not explicitly noted in Case 4.1, an awareness that the two communities were heavily impacted by social conditions (e.g., poverty, lack of services). From a CG EBP perspective, Tiempo de Oro recognized and respected the different communication formats that were present (Spanish, English, and the Pascua Yaqui languages); the different decision-making processes and customs that were at work; and the normative expectations as to how relationships are to be appropriately established and maintained over time. Additionally, Tiempo de Oro's culturally attuned prevention–intervention strategy followed accepted community engagement techniques as described in the literature. The process began by contacting the key gatekeepers of the target communities (Florio & Raschko, 1998); *ElderVention*, 1997).

A Quantitative Look at the Tiempo de Oro Prevention Intervention

Alongside its qualitative assessments, Tiempo de Oro applied an array of outcome measures to track its CG-EBP-oriented intervention. The first arm of the program's intervention encompassed community education presentations, which were monitored using pre- and postpresentation questionnaires that were administered verbally by prevention specialists in the field. Subsequently, the Tiempo de Oro evaluator conducted a meta-analysis of all presentations for which complete data could be obtained. El Mirage yielded 39 presentations for which reliable prepost data were obtained, and Guadalupe yielded 28 presentations. The number of correct answers on the pretest was matched with the number of correct posttest answers for each presentation. Using two arrays (pretest versus posttest for matched subject groups), a t test showed a pretest mean of 20.82 at El Mirage and a posttest mean of 25.79. The SPSS t score was −5.41, with a significance level at .001 (two tailed). The Guadalupe pretests had a mean of 39.07 and a posttest mean of 50.50. The SPSS t score was −4.05, with a significance level at .001 (two tailed). The findings indicate that the participants were significantly more knowledgeable about risk factors after the presentations than before them. From a program evaluation standpoint, Tiempo de Oro has shown that its culturally attuned community-based behavioral and mental health directed presentations are demonstrating effectiveness relative to increasing participant knowledge.

The second element of Tiempo de Oro's intervention protocol was its *workshops*, (the support group–topical prevention intervention format), whose outcomes were tracked using the Life Satisfaction Index (LSI; Neugarten, Havinghurst, & Tobin, 1961). This interventive modality likewise shows similar positive outcome trends. It should be noted that the LSI is closer to a trait-type measure (Stock, Okun, & Benin, 1986) and functions best if a longer time interval is allowed between administrations because one would not expect great change after each individual workshop, but, rather, after a participant had been exposed to a cluster of workshop sessions. For the purposes of a preliminary analysis, the participants were divided into "low exposure" (four or fewer workshop sessions, $n = 25$) and "high exposure" (five or more workshop sessions, $n = 26$). An SPSS t test was performed on each group. Results showed that the high exposure ($n = 26$) LSI pretest mean was 14.69, while the posttest mean was 17.00. The t score was -2.745 and statistical significance was at the .01 level ($p \leq .01$). In the low exposure ($n = 25$) group, the LSI pretest mean was 15.44 and the posttest mean was 18.52. The t score was -4.314 and the statistical significance was at the .01 level ($p \leq .01$). It is important to note that even the low-exposure group registered positive outcomes.

The third element of Tiempo de Oro's program was its *home visits* to less mobile seniors with the intent to reduce levels of social isolation, depression, and suicidal ideation. Here the outcomes were tracked using Section D of the Government Performance and Reporting Act (GPRA) instrument, a uniformly required instrument for all nine PARC TCE sites. The subscale comprised questions 2–9 (question 4 excepted) on the GPRA. These questions related directly or indirectly to self-report of vegetative or cognitive symptoms of depression. The program evaluator obtained 28 sets of client data with complete intake and six-month follow-up data. Subscale data derived at intake were labeled "pretests" and the six-month follow-up data were considered "posttests." An SPSS matched pair t test was preformed (two tailed). The pretest mean was 12.53 and the posttest mean was 9.28. The t score was 3.12 with a significance of $p \leq .01$. From a program evaluation standpoint, the home visits can be effective in decreasing participants' reported depressive symptoms.

Group CBT Focused Treatment and Rural Loners: A CG EBP Qualitative Overview

The second PARC Partner Site participating in the CG EBP effort was the Health Improvement Program for the Elderly, a four-agency collaboration, led by Jewish Family and Children's Services. The collaborative agreed on cognitive behavioral therapy (CBT) as it choice for it EBP intervention. CBT allowed the therapists to provide their treatments in several modes (i.e., individual, home-based, or group therapy sessions) to a number of subpopulations including Holocaust survivors, grandparents raising grandchildren, and individuals living in rural to remote areas of Pima County. These latter encompassed mostly Euro ethnic heritage residents of the rural community of Marana 25 miles northwest of Tucson. An increasing need for mental and behavioral health services had emerged among the Marana residents who had aged in place. Some of these residents had been in Marana for much of their adult lives on small farms, raised children, and seen them move away; others arrived in their middle years and were continuing to live in their often dated trailers, which were less accommodating to the older owners. All not only lived some distance from the Marana Valley primary health-care clinic (a 15 to 30 minute drive), but also were a substantial distance from acute and residential care resources in Tucson, a 30 to 45 minute drive. From a cultural perspective, these residents were staying on by choice and were living as disparate individuals in the extreme isolation of a harsh desert environment. However, they were also facing their increasing frailties while nonetheless trying to hold onto their preferred loner lifestyles and outlooks.

CASE 4.2A: ENGAGING AND SERVING CLIENTS IN A RURAL SETTING—ESTABLISHING INDIVIDUAL CBT CONTACT

The Marana community presents a seemingly pastoral image. This is especially so if one enters Marana Valley after passing through the strikingly beautiful desert national forest containing the 30–40-foot Suhuaro cactus trees. Coming from this direction, one arrives at a very spread out and sparsely populated Southwestern rural area where people have either come to settle as loners, or who now find themselves as loners, having aged in place.

Marana has been Jack Prohaska's regular professional beat for some time now, working out of the behavioral health unit at the Marana Community Health Center, one of the four Health Improvement for the Elderly demonstration project partner agencies. We spoke about Mr. C., a crusty, 82-year-old, Euro Anglo ex-house painter who had settled in Marana at his retirement some 30 years before. Even though he had lived alone during most of this period, he had maintained links to family and friends. However, these contacts had broken off. About two years earlier than the present contact, he developed a serious respiratory infection, which set in as a chronic condition. To add to the problem, he had returned to his old smoking habit. Periodically, he would come into the Marana Community Health Center with acute respiratory inflammation. This pattern continued over a year with no improvement. Nothing seemed to work, particularly with regard to stopping Mr. C's smoking. The primary care physician and behavioral health unit staffed his case and developed an intervention plan. Mr. C. was told that he had a weak respiratory system, but it was controllable at home— if he stopped smoking. He was told that a behavioral health approach might help. He had been resistant to using behavioral health services. Mr. C. was also told his actual prognosis, namely, that the next respiratory inflammatory episode would most likely land him in the hospital (30 miles away) and from there he might need to be in a convalescent facility (rather than return to his Marana home).

Mr. C. acquiesced to have a behavioral health session but did not agree to stop smoking. Enter Jack. He immediately recognized that counseling alone, even combined with the threat of hospitalization was not enough. However, a treatment clue emerged within the counseling conversation. Mr. C. admitted that he liked to smoke because he had nothing else that was fun in his life. Jack knew enough of the community to remember that over the last decade Mr. C. appeared to have lost contact with all his family and friends, and so he set out to repair Mr. C's network. He arranged for family members still in the greater Tucson area to reestablish contact. He also got him in touch with some friends. It has been a complete year now. Mr. C. has stopped smoking and there have been no further acute respiratory problems. Although still not overly talkative about himself, Mr. C. has nonetheless admitted to Jack that his days "are pretty full now."

The treatment plan described in Case 4.2a combining CBT treatment and a very pragmatic social-network intervention worked. But then this is the way Jack carried out his practice, whether these fixes included mobilizing resources to refit old trailers with access ramps for the now wheelchair-bound elderly or reestablishing their friendship networks. However, the need for a more effective use of staff time and resources relative to the increased demand for services also surfaced. Group-focused CBT was seen as a potential solution. But here the Health Improvement Program therapists ran into another aspect of the Marana Valley cultural norms. Jack Prohaska and Virginia Cappeller, the Health Improvement Program clinical director, wanted to experiment with a CBT group support effort. The problem was how to develop acceptance of the group approach among persons not valuing therapy groups.

CASE 4.2B: ESTABLISHING A CBT THERAPY GROUP FOR RURAL LONERS

The success with Mr. C. brought a new problem to the surface. There were a number of Marana clinic clients like him, with similar health problems and social interaction deficits, for whom the conventional counseling intervention strategy alone was having limited success. Jack had long recognized the potential effectiveness of and the need for group therapy sessions. However, his early overtures to several clients to form a treatment group had been rebuffed. But as Jack stood back and looked anew at the problem, he noted that although still outwardly a loner, Mr. C. had begun to relish another suggested activity: attending occasional lunches at the senior center. At Jack's suggestion, a novel tactic was employed. Since it was the time for the Clinic's annual service plan review, he proposed that, instead of the usual client surveys, the several elderly clients with need profiles similar to Mr. C.'s be invited to a "focus group session" in which discussion would take place and refreshments served. The "talk and cookies" session was a hit. The loner-oriented clients found the group experience rewarding, to the extent that they asked for more regular meetings. With the original focus group content completed, the members began to discuss community problems, and from there their own needs. A CBT focus was presented to and accepted by the group members. These group therapy sessions have continued, with faithful attendance by the original members who, in turn, have invited others of their acquaintances to participate. Additionally, the group members are not in the least adverse to periodically turning a session, or part of a session into a "focus group" activity to make suggestions to the Marana Valley Clinic around improving and extending services.

The treatment strategies described in the cases involved careful maneuvering through several layers of embedded cultural outlooks. From the CG EBP context, it was not only the client cultures that needed the cultural attention, but also those of the provider organizations that needed to modify their approaches. As described earlier (see Figure 4.1), it is not just the clients or participants who bring their culture with them into the intervention, but the providers, managers, and line staff also come with their preferences and value orientations (in this case, CBT formatted for individual and group formats). The key staff members used their culturally grounded knowledge of the service environment and came up with a normatively acceptable strategy. While the elderly loners were resistant to the idea of group therapy, they were attracted to the focus group process. This group experience, although initiated for a different purpose, proved so satisfying that they asked for a second session, and from there additional regular meetings that had a more personal problem-identifying and problem-solving emphasis. The acceptance of the CBT group intervention was related to the clients buying into the experience in terms of their own perceived benefits, as well as their willingness to abate their own loner status, in favor of more regular social support received in group therapy sessions.

The application of several CG EBP operational principles can be observed. As outlined in Figure 4.1, the practitioners were dealing with two different cultural perceptual systems, the rural loners and the Health Improvement Program's behavioral health orientations. Although resistant to considering himself as being in therapy, Mr. C. liked the idea of having his social networks reestablished. As for the group treatment, the Marana elderly residents had to first experience the benefits of having a good time and discovering what Guberman and Maheu (2004) point to as the similarities of their situations, before engaging in problem solving and counseling. The common ground may not be based on complete value changes or even reorientations, but, rather, accommodations that are made around converging or commonly agreed upon goals (Jecker, Carrese, & Pearlman, 1995).

The Quantitative Side of the Health Improvement Program for the Elderly Intervention

As two of its principal outcome measures, the Health Improvement Program for the Elderly employed the State/Trait Anxiety Scale (Spielberger, 1989) and the Geriatric Depression Scale (GDS; Yesavage, 1988). Client records were maintained on the Web-based data management system (previously described); data were entered from remote sites readying it for immediate analysis. Analyses were conducted to determine if there were significant differences among the clients at baseline and six months after entering treatment. As summarized in Table 4.1, preliminary outcome assessment results show a positive direction between baseline and six months posttreatment.

Several other outcome variables—difficulties with managing activities of daily living, level of apathy, and overall perceived health status—likewise moved in a positive direction (see Table 4.2).

The data are also yielding some potential variations between the study populations. As of this writing, 241 clients have been served with the Euro ethnic subgroup accounting for 199, or 82.6%, and the Latinos for 42, or 17.4%, of the sample. Some of the differences that are emerging center around such factors as daily coping activities, with Latinos needing more

TABLE 4.1   Paired T Test of State/Trait Anxiety and Depression

	State Anxiety ($n = 85$)	Trait Anxiety ($n = 84$)	Depression ($n = 81$)
Pre	47.93 ± 12.3	47.23 ± 11.8	7.74 ± 3.5
Post	42.34 ± 13.6	42.85 ± 11.6	5.06 ± 3.3
df	84	83	80
t value	3.735	3.873	6.787
p value	$< .001$	$< .000$	$< .000$

TABLE 4.2   Paired *T* Test of Difficulty Managing Daily Needs, Apathy, and Overall Health

	Difficulty With Managing Daily Needs (*n* = 130)	Difficulty With Apathy (*n* = 130	Overall Health (*n* = 130)
Pre	2.86 ± 1.64	2.74 ± 1.42	2.28 ± 1.12
Post	2.44 ± 1.88	2.03 ± 1.33	2.48 ± 1.08
df	129	129	129
t value	2.761	4.188	−2.337
p value	.007	.000	.021

assistance with using the telephone to access service systems (X^2 = 3.75, df = 1, *p* = .05) and help with environmental barriers (X^2 = 5.41, df = 1, *p* = .02); they also had more learning barriers (X^2 = 5.37, df = 1, *p* = .02). Additionally, Latinos reported more emotional barriers in using the Health Improvement Program's treatment processes (X^2 = 5.60, df = 1, *p* = .02), indicated higher levels of cultural barriers (X^2 = 8.78, df = 1, *p* = .003), and registered higher GDS scores at baseline (X^2 = 2.70, df = 74, *p* = .009).

The Health Improvement Program for the elderly is also pursuing a longitudinal analysis of the construct of social support, both in the Marana Valley and with the Tucson metropolitan clients. The program therapists see themselves as facilitating the social reengagement of their elderly clients (Cattan, Newell, Bond, & White, 2003) and make referrals to social activities in addition to the application of CBT.

IMPLEMENTATION, DOCUMENTATION, MEASUREMENT, AND OUTCOME ISSUES

Two major questions arise with regard to the implementation of CG EBP: (1) What goes into designing and implementing a CG EBP effort? (2) How do you measure the culturally grounded component of the practice and subsequently link such measurements to the EBP effort?

Designing and Implementing a CG EBP Effort

The core elements of the CG EBP design were first assembled within the proposals that were funded at the PARC TCE Partner Sites. These efforts were complemented by the introduction of the conceptual framework by the PARC

TCE (as outlined in the earlier section, The Conceptual Base) and shared through the PARC coaching connection. From the start, the CG and EBP approaches were understood as necessary and complementary to each other. With regard to the cultural aspects of their programs, the Partner Sites maintained the following three ongoing information-gathering, information-upgrading, and catchment area networking steps:

1. Gathering detailed information about their target catchment areas, and their multicultural client/participant populations, along with their changing demographics as they aged in place.
2. Connecting with the communicational and relational infrastructure of the community settings and environments where the clients and participants resided.
3. Linking to the available provider infrastructure while keeping in mind the need to make referrals and linkages that would be culturally appropriate to the client population.

With regard to sustaining the EBP integrity of their respective interventions, the Partner Sites followed the steps outlined in SAMHSA's guide to science-based practices (*Science-Based,* 2001) whose principal elements included:

- The interventions in both their cultural and EBP components were theory based and operational model driven.
- There were standardization of measures, data collection, and data analysis, employing both accepted statistical techniques and proven qualitative evaluation methods.
- Attention was given to both the fidelity to the intervention methodologies and documenting any adaptations.
- There was ongoing monitoring of the interventions in order to incorporate new information and enhance practitioner practice.
- Outcome assessments were woven into the fabric of the interventions, with the intent of providing useful quantitative and qualitative information to the field.

Figure 4.3 provides a summary of the full range of the organizational components that need to be considered in culturally grounded and evidence-based interventions. For example, the Partner Sites provided considerable time and effort to the interorganizational (fellow provider) environments. The Site leaders recognized that information and referral assistance does not just happen, but requires working relationships with other providers. Likewise, CG EBP attention was necessary in the broader policy and funding

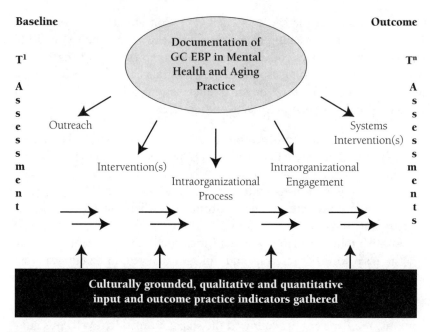

FIGURE 4.3   Overview of organization-wide CG EBP implementation.

systems to which the Arizona Sites related. Culturally attuned inputs were made and tracked at all levels and at both the preliminary and ongoing stages of the overall CG EBP effort, however, the discussion here has focused on the direct practice aspects of CG EBP.

Measuring CG and Linking to EBP

Nine variables that are crucial for CG EBP to flourish were identified. The scales and measures suggested in Figures 4.4 and 4.5 result from observations about how the Partner Sites designed and conducted their EBP projects with culturally, generationally, and regionally diverse populations. They represent the basic cultural knowledge and practice skills expected of the EBP practitioner. Figure 4.4 presents these nine variables in the context of the practitioner's *cultural knowledge* capabilities.

Variables 1, 2, 3, 4, and 9 in Figure 4.4 flow directly from the conceptual model discussed in the earlier section, The Conceptual Base. For example, in their initial proposals, in their work plans, and in their staff training and supervision, the Partner Site leadership expected their field staff to be familiar with the specific *demographic profiles* of the target populations (variable 1 in Figure 4.4). Likewise, the staff were expected to be knowledgeable

Culturally Attuned Knowledge Variables	Ratings					Qualitative Comments
	1	2	3	4	5	
1. Group demographics	1	2	3	4	5	_____
2. Communication patterns	1	2	3	4	5	_____
3. Customs	1	2	3	4	5	_____
4. Norms, values, and beliefs	1	2	3	4	5	_____
5. Acculturation factors	1	2	3	4	5	_____
6. Active listening	1	2	3	4	5	_____
7. Rapport building	1	2	3	4	5	_____
8. Help seeking and accepting	1	2	3	4	5	_____
9. Socioeconomic, status, etc., confounds, sorted out	1	2	3	4	5	_____

Practitioner ratings: 1-no knowledge, 2-little knowledge, 3-basic knowledge, 4-advanced knowledge, 5-comprehensive knowledge (based on *demonstration* knowledge).

FIGURE 4.4   CG EBP Cultural Knowledge Rating Scale (CKRS).

about the *ethnic language preferences* or the *local idiomatic expressions* used by the populations in their day-to-day communications (variable 2). Additionally, staff were expected to be knowledgeable of local *cultural customs* and *courtesies* (variable 3). The cultural knowledge expectations extended also to staff knowledge and understanding of the target group member's *value outlooks* and *belief systems* (variable 4), especially in the areas of mental and behavioral health concerns and around the issues of counseling or therapy, all of which retain a residual popular culture stigma (Chen, Kramer, Chen, & Chung, 2005; Graham et al., 2003; Scheffer, 2003; Marwaha & Livingston, 2002). Additionally the Partner Site leadership expected their intervention staff to be knowledgeable about *socioeconomic and other status factors* (variable 9) influencing the target populations.

Through the coaching observations, several other cultural knowledge capabilities emerged. It became clear that the Partner Site leadership expected staff to understand how acculturation factors played themselves out with their respective populations (variable 5) along with the roles that culturally attuned *active listening* (variable 6) and *rapport building* (variable 7) play when one is engaging another person *across* cultures. These added requirements of culturally attuned active listening and culturally attuned rapport building became standard components of the training and supervisory content provided by the Partner Site leadership. Finally, the Partner Sites identified the need to recognize the cultural overlays around *help-seeking* and *help-accepting* orientations (variable 8) to the practitioners CG EBP capabilities (Valle, 1998).

Measuring the Practice Skills Requirement Component of CG EBP

A practitioner must not only have the knowledge of what constitutes a reputable CG EBP intervention but must also be skilled in applying this knowledge. The Partner Site leadership required their staff not just to know about their target populations, but to also be able to engage their clients around the client's cultural norms and customs. Moreover, the Partner Sites expected their staff to be able identify both *between* and *within* cultural group differences and similarities in order to avoid working from cultural stereotypes. Figure 4.5 presents the same set of culturally grounded variables outlined in Figure 4.4, but that the focus is on the cross-cultural skills of the practitioner.

A Further Step: Developing Cultural Knowledge and Skill Indicators

The observations of the cultural practices at the Partner Sites yielded additional information about the cultural expertise needed in EBP practice. For example, the Partner Site leaders would focus on a specific cultural practice *variable*, drawing their own particular list of practice events, or *indicators*, that they knew were directly linked to a specific cultural practice variable. If the known target population was a Latino elderly group, the list of indicators was longer than just noting if the preferred language was Spanish. The list also included such details as to whether the preferred communication pattern was face-to-face, by phone, and so on. Other types of indicator details included the extent of formality expected from a younger person or from a stranger when addressing an elder, or whether the communication should take place in the client's home or in a local community setting (with the latter providing more privacy from family or neighbors). Alertness to the nonverbal communications was likewise expected (e.g., whether to sit or stand

Culturally Attuned Skills Variables	Ratings 1	2	3	4	5	Qualitative Comments
1. Group demographics	1	2	3	4	5	_____
2. Communication patterns	1	2	3	4	5	_____
3. Customs	1	2	3	4	5	_____
4. Norms, values, and beliefs	1	2	3	4	5	_____
5. Acculturation factors	1	2	3	4	5	_____
6. Active listening	1	2	3	4	5	_____
7. Rapport building	1	2	3	4	5	_____
8. Help seeking and accepting	1	2	3	4	5	_____
9. Socioeconomic, status, etc., confounds, sorted out	1	2	3	4	5	_____

Practitioner ratings: 1-no knowledge, 2-little knowledge, 3-basic knowledge, 4-advanced knowledge, 5-comprehensive knowledge (based on *evidenced* knowledge).

FIGURE 4.5   CG EBP Cultural Skills Rating Scale (CSRS).

if an elder walks into the room, the expected behaviors around shaking hands, the proximity with which strangers stand near each other). Additionally, it was observed that the Partner Site leadership also wanted to know if the field staff was attuned to the cultural art décor of the home and other visibly displayed cultural symbols.

Figure 4.6 provides a potentially replicable approach to specifying indicators for specific variables. The example in Figure 4.6 relates to variable 4, the normative expectations and beliefs around depression, in both Figures 4.4 and 4.5. The example examines how some more traditionally oriented Latinos might look at CBT treatment for depression, and it identifies indicators that the practitioner could use to illustrate how less acculturated and more traditional Latino subgroup members might look at such treatment.

In Figure 4.6, the CG EBP expectation would center on the practitioner's ability to (a) recognize the extent of *stigma* around a mental health

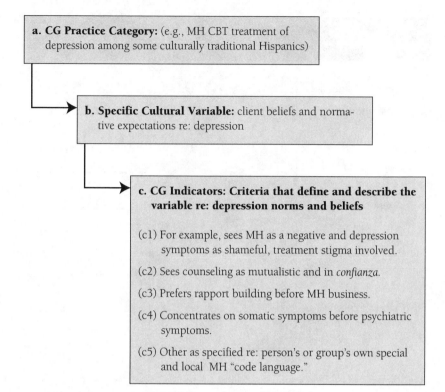

FIGURE 4.6   Measuring culturally grounded CG EBP: Establishing specific operational indicators.

intervention relative to a specific Latino cohort (item c1); (b) engage in counseling as a *confianza* (a mutualistic exchange) experience (item c2) instead of as a professional–client distancing format; (c) deal with the normative expectation that the intervention would first focus on *rapport building* rather than on establishing treatment objectives or a treatment contract (item c3); (d) recognize that the more traditional culture-oriented Hispanic elder client might focus more on somatic (behavioral health) factors than on more cognitive or possibly affective symptomatology (item c4); and (e) understand and sanction the use of the client's preferred terminology in contrast to the more biomedical or technical mental and behavioral health terminology (item c5).

From a PARC coaching observational standpoint, the detailing of the rating scales in both Figures 4.4 and 4.5 simply make more explicit the actual supervisory techniques of Partner Site managers, while the cultural practice indicators in Figure 4.6 illustrate the types of specific practitioner behaviors that actually serve to operationalize each of the nine identified CG EBP variables.

LESSONS LEARNED AND THE DISTANCE YET TO GO

The figures in this chapter provide an outline through which to examine the CG EBP effort as well as to summarize the pathways taken. Figure 4.1 describes the fundamental understandings with which the PARC TCE Partner Sites approached their respective CG EBP interventions. Mental and behavioral health services bring their cultural perspective with them, as does the EBP field, as do the diverse clients in these services. Different sets of culturally influenced rules and expectations are at work for the provider and the consumer alike. Additionally, these rules and expectations (i.e., the cultural dynamics at work) are more often than not implicit rather than explicit. In an EBP context, it is the task of the practitioner to make the cultural dynamics as explicit as possible. In their initial proposals, the Partner Sites prepared themselves for this eventuality, as did the PARC TCE through its coaching process.

Figure 4.2 illustrates the manner in which PARC and the Partner Sites, using the CG EBP framework, set out to appropriately distinguish between cultural and social status domain variables relative to their respective diverse elderly ethnic populations. It also highlights the need to employ both qualitative and quantitative documentation efforts in order to provide the full context of the cultural dimensions of the practice.

Figure 4.3 summarizes how the PARC TCE Partner Sites each worked internally with their own parent organization, and externally within the interorganizational environment to both mobilize and sustain support for the total CG EBP effort over time. The figure also illustrates that launching and maintaining a CG EBP intervention effort is more than just hiring a few culturally capable staff, or relegating the effort to a portion of a program. It is an organization-wide enterprise and must remain so if it is to succeed.

Figures 4.4, 4.5, and 4.6 bring the focus back to the central issue in this discussion, namely, how CG EBP is to be measured within an EBP context. As noted earlier, the nine CG EBP variables identified in Figures 4.4 and 4.5 emerged from the combination of available theory and the direct observation of the Partner Site cultural practices. The examples of the operational indicators in Figure 4.6 and the accompanying discussion of other possible indicators are further refinements of these observations. Collectively, the CG EBP effort reported here provides a starting point for the measurement of the cultural components of EBP.

Some Recognized Limitations

The cultural knowledge and practice skills rating scales (Figures 4.4 and 4.5) and the variable indicators (Figure 4.6) all constitute practices as observed rather than instruments that have been tested. The variables enumerated in the scales do reflect the distillation of the process information described. However, more work is needed. In this context, the nine-variables frameworks of key expected cultural knowledge and skills and their accompanying indicators are offered as preliminary suggestions as to how to proceed with the empirical documentation of culturally attuned practice. Additionally, it is important to note that CG EBP remains in the middle ground of the evidentiary work undertaken to demonstrate viable mechanisms for integrating culture into EBP. At this writing, CG EBP is more sharply defined than basic mental health practice, but there is still a distance to go to empirically define the complete attributes of *cultural competency* in EBP. CG EBP as described herein presents a good start, but it is only a start. This limitation is summarized in Figure 4.7.

In Conclusion

The expressed need to account for the role of cultural factors within mental health has a long history (Whaley, 2003; Karno, 1966). This need now extends to the EBP arena (Ruiz, 2004; Williams 2004). Fortunately, the SAMHSA TCE initiative being reported here allowed for the documentation

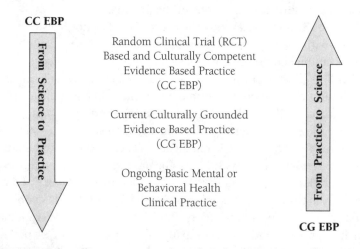

FIGURE 4.7   Culturally competent evidence-based practice (CC EBP): Strategic considerations. (*Source:* Positive Aging Resource Center, 2004.)

of applied cultural strategies in behavioral and mental health services for ethnically, generationally, and regionally diverse elderly. This funding provided the opportunity for both the PARC TCE and its Partner Sites to field test the specific culturally attuned approaches as they were implemented within actual multicultural community-based settings. From the start, the Partner Sites geared up their respective programs to implement the CG EBP strategy in concert with their distinct missions. The PARC TCE, through its coaching mechanism, provided both the support and the observational technology. As Bartels et al. (2002, p. 1428) indicate,

> Evidence-based practice is based on careful and appropriate use of the findings from the best relevant studies, accompanied by the limits of the existing data. In some instances the best studies include randomized controlled trials, whereas in other situations, nonrandomized outcome studies or case reports may constitute the best evidence base.

The undertaking reported here is a nonrandomized case report in need of further verification. The challenge that now faces the EBP field is specifically how to take *culturally grounded* EBP to the next level of *culturally competent* EBP, employing a rigorous testing strategy. Brach and Fraser (2000) suggest that culturally competent practitioners can reduce the access and treatment disparities encountered by ethnically diverse populations. Culture is a filter through which cognition, affect, and behavior flow. And it is the practitioner's ability to identify and work through this filtering process that is the core of cultural competence. Moreover, it is a working understanding of this filtering process that assists in extinguishing the debilitating impact of *cultural stereotypes* that van Ryn and Fu (2003) identify as permeating current practice with culturally diverse populations. This paper as a whole provides an outline of how to proceed. CG EBP has demonstrated its utility as the means whereby the practitioner can identify the true heterogeneity present in the multicultural social environment. Miranda et al. (2005, p. 134) highlight what they identify as "two areas of [mental health] research needing immediate attention":

> First, methodologies for tailoring evidence-based interventions for specific populations would be extremely helpful. Because culture is continuously evolving, the ability to identify factors that are amenable to adaptation, while maintaining the critical ingredients of care, would provide a methodology for continually ensuring that care is sensitive to the needs and concerns of any client group. Second, although beyond the scope of this review, we would be remiss in noting that ethnic minorities are less likely to receive mental health care, than are majority populations.

To the list of those populations less likely to receive mental health care we would also add the elderly and the rural and isolated populations discussed in this chapter. In our view, therefore, the CG EBP effort reported provides a feasible starting point for infusing cultural considerations into EBP as called for by Miranda et al. (2005). The door has been opened to further culturally guided practice research. These next steps now await future priority attention by both funders and the EBP field. A commitment of resources and an investment of time is needed.

ACKNOWLEDGEMENT

The comprehensive editing assistance by Kristine Stilwell, PhD, with regard to both the format and the substance of this discussion is most gratefully acknowledged.

REFERENCES

Areán, P. A., Cook, B. L., Gallagher-Thompson, D., Hegel M. T., Schulberg, H. C., & Schulz, R. (2003). Guidelines for conducting geropsychotherapy research. *Journal of Geriatric Psychiatry, 11,* 9–16.

Bartels, S. J., Dums, A. R., Oxman, T. E., Schneider, L. S., Areán, P. A., Alexopoulus, G. S., et al. (2002). Evidence based practices in geriatric mental health care. *Psychiatric Services, 53,* 1419–1431.

Beiser, M. (2003). Why should we care about culture? *Canadian Journal of Psychiatry, 48,* 154–160.

Bernal, G., & Scharrón-del-Río, M. R. (2001). Are empirically supported treatments valid for ethnic minorities? Toward an alternative approach for treatment research. *Cultural Diversity and Ethnic Minority Psychology, 7,* 328–342.

Borson, S., Bartels, S. J., Colenda, C. C., Gottleib, G. L., & Meyers, B. (2001). Geriatric mental health services research: A strategic plan for an aging population. *American Journal of Geriatric Psychiatry, 9,* 191–204.

Brach, C., & Fraser, I. (2000). Can cultural competency reduce racial and ethnic health disparities? A review and conceptual model. *Medical Care Research and Review, 57*(Suppl 1), 181–227.

Cattan, M., Newell, C., Bond, J., & White, M. (2003). Alleviating social isolation and loneliness among older people. *International Journal of Mental Health, 5,* 20–30.

Chambless, D. L., Baker, M. J., Baucom, D. H., Beutler, L. E., Calhoun, K. S., Crits-Cristoph, P. (1998). Update on empirically validated therapies, II. *The Clinical Psychologist, 51,* 3–16.

Chen, H., Kramer, E. J., Chen, T., & Chung, H. (2005). Engaging Asian Americans for mental health research: Challenges and solutions. *Journal of Immigrant Health, 7,* 109–116.

Dilworth-Anderson, P., & Gibson, B. E. (2002). The cultural influence of values, norms, meanings, and perceptions in understanding dementia in ethnic minorities. *Alzheimer Disease and Associated Disorders, 16*(Suppl 2), S56–S63.

ElderVention: First year evaluation and summary, July 1996–June 1997. (1997). Phoenix, AZ: Area Agency on Aging, Inc.

Evidence-based practices: An implementation guide for community-based substance abuse treatment agencies. (2003). Iowa City, IA: The Iowa Consortium for Substance Abuse Research and Evaluation.

Florio, E. R., & Raschko, R. (1998). The gatekeeper model: Implications for social policy, *Journal of Aging & Social Policy, 10,* 37–55.

Gerrish, K., & Clayton, J. (2004). Promoting evidence-based practice: An organizational approach. *Journal of Nursing Management, 12,* 114–113.

Gittell, R., & Vidal, A. (1998). *Community organizing: Building social capital as a development strategy.* Thousand Oaks, CA: Sage Publications.

Goldman, H. H., Thelander, S., & Cleas-Goran, W. (2000). Organizing mental health services: An evidence-based approach. *Journal of Mental Health Policy and Economics, 3,* 69–75.

Graham, N., Lindesay, J., Katona, C., Bertolote, J. M., Camus, V., Copeland, J. R. M., et al. (2003). Reducing stigma and discrimination against older people with mental disorders: A technical consensus statement. *International Journal of Geriatric Psychiatry, 18,* 670–678.

Guarnaccia, P. J., Martinez, I., & Acosta, H. (2002). *Comprehensive in-depth literature review and analysis of Hispanic mental health issues.* Mercerville, NJ: New Jersey Mental Health Institute, Inc.

Guidelines for providers of psychological services to ethnic, linguistic, and culturally diverse populations. (1993). *American Psychologist, 48,* 45–48.

Guterman, A., & Miller, I. (1989). The influence of the organization on clinical practice. *Clinical Social Work Journal, 12,* 151–163.

Health Literacy. (1999). Report of the Council on Scientific Affairs, *Journal of the American Medical Association, 281,* 552–557.

Jecker, N. S., Carrese, J. A., & Pearlman, R. A. (1995). Caring for patients in cross-cultural settings. *Hastings Center Report, 25,* 6–14.

Kaestle, C. F., Campbell, A., Finn, J. D., Johnson, S. T., Mikulecky, J. L. (2001). *Adult literacy and education in America.* Washington, DC: U.S. Department of Education, Office of Educational Research and Improvement, NCES 2001-534.

Karno, M. (1966). The enigma of ethnicity in a psychiatric clinic. *Archives of General Psychiatry, 14,* 516–520.

Lambert, D., Donahue, J. D., Mitchell, M., & Strauss, R. (2003). *Rural mental health outreach: Promising practices in rural areas.* Washington, DC: U.S. Department of Health and Human Services; Substance Abuse and Mental Health Services Administration, Center for Mental Health Services.

Lau, A. W., & Gallagher-Thompson, D. (2002). Ethnic minority older adults in clinical and research programs: Issues and recommendations. *Behavior Therapist, 25*(1), 10–11, 16.

Levkoff, S. E., Levy, B. R., & Weitzman, P. F. (2000). The matching model of recruitment. *Journal of Mental Health and Aging, 6,* 29–38.

Levkoff, S. E., & Sanchez, H. (2003). Lessons learned about minority recruitment from the Centers on Minority Aging and Health Promotion. In L. Curry & J. Jackson (Eds.), *The science of inclusion: Recruiting and retaining racial and ethnic elders in health research* (pp. 8–16). Washington, DC: Gerontological Society of America.

Li, R. M., McCardle, P., Clark, R. L., Kinsella, K., & Berch, D. (2001). *Diverse voices: The inclusion of language-minority populations in national studies: Challenges and opportunities.* Washington, DC: National Institute on Aging, National Institute of Child Health and Human Development, National Center on Minority Health and Health Disparities.

Marwaha, S., & Livingston, G. (2002). Stigma, racism, or choice: Why do depressed ethnic elders avoid psychiatrists. *Journal of Affective Disorders,* 257–262.

McDonel Herr, E., English, M. J., & Brown, N. B. (2003). Translating mental health services research into practice: A perspective from staff at the US Substance Abuse and Mental Health Services Administration. *Alzheimer's Care Quarterly,* 241–252.

Miranda, J., Azocar, F., Organista, K. C., Muñoz, R. F., & Lieberman, A. (1996). Recruiting and retaining low-income Latinos in psychotherapy research. *Journal of Counseling and Clinical Psychology, 64,* 868–874.

Miranda, J., Bernal, G., Lau, A., Kohn, L., Hwang, W.-C., & LaFromboise, T. (2005). State of science on psychosocial interventions for ethnic minorities. *Annual Review of Clinical Psychology, 1,* 113–142.

Miranda, J., Nakamura, R., & Bernal, G. (2003). Including ethnic minorities in mental health intervention research: A practical approach to a long standing problem. *Culture, Medicine, and Psychiatry, 27,* 467–486.

Montoro-Rodriguez, J., Kosloski, K., & Montgomery, R. J. V. (2003). Evaluating a practice-oriented service model to increase the use of respite services among minorities and rural caregivers. *Gerontologist, 43,* 916–924.

Neugarten, B. L., Havinghurst, R. J, & Tobin, S. (1961). The measurement of life satisfaction. *Journal of Gerontology, 16,* 134–143.

Pinn, V. W. (2003). From policy to science: Enhancing the inclusion of diverse ethnic groups in aging research. In L. Curry & J. Jackson (Eds.), *The science of inclusion: Recruiting and retaining racial and ethnic elders in health research* (pp. 1–7). Washington, DC: Gerontological Society of America.

Review of minority aging research at the NIA, Executive Summary. Accessed September 27, 2004.

Rogler, L. H., Malgady, R. G., Costantino, G., & Blumenthal. (1987). What do culturally sensitive mental health services mean: The case of Hispanics. *American Psychologist, 42,* 565–570.

Ruiz, P. (2004). Culture, race and ethnicity in psychiatric practice. *Psychiatric Annals, 34,* 527–532.

Scheffer, R. (2003). Addressing stigma: Increasing public understanding of mental illness. Presented to the Standing Committee on Social Affairs, Science, and Technology, Washington DC.

Science-based substance abuse prevention: A guide. (2001). Rockville, MD: Substance Abuse and Mental Health Services Administration, Center for Substance Abuse Prevention, Division of Knowledge Development and Evaluation. Retrieved from www.samhsa.gov.

Spielberger, C. D. (1989). *State-trait anxiety inventory: A comprehensive biography.* Palo Alto, CA: Consulting Psychologists Press.

Stock, W. A., Okun, M. A., & Benin, M. (1986). Structure of subjective well-being among the elderly. *Psychology and Aging, 1,* 91–102.

Tseng, W.-S., & Streltzer, J. (Eds.). (2001). *Culture and psychotherapy: A guide to clinical practice.* Washington, DC: American Psychiatric Publishing Inc.

Unequal treatment: Confronting racial and ethnic disparities in health care. (2002). Washington, DC: Institute of Medicine, National Academy Press.

Valle, R. (1988–1989). Outreach to ethnic minorities with Alzheimer's disease: The challenge to the community. *Health Matrix, 6,* 13–27.

Valle, R. (1998). *Caregiving across cultures: Working with dementing illness and ethnically diverse populations.* Washington, DC: Taylor and Francis.

van Ryn, M., & Fu, S. S. (2003). Paved with good intentions: Do public health and human service providers contribute to racial/ethnic disparities in health? *American Journal of Public Health, 93,* 248–255.

Whaley, A. L. (2003). Ethnicity/race, ethics, and epidemiology. *Journal of the National Medical Association, 95,* 736–742.

Williams, D. R. (2003). Racism and health. In K. E. Whitfield (Ed.), *Closing the gap: Improving the health of minority elders in the new millennium* (pp. 69–79). Washington, DC: Gerontological Society of America.

Williams, R. (2004). Evidence into practice: The culture and context of modern professionalism in psychiatry. *Current Opinion in Psychiatry, 17,* 237–242.

Yesavage, J. A. (1988). Geriatric depression scale (short form). *Psychopharmacology Bulletin, 24,* 709–711.

CHAPTER 5

Evidence-Based Practices for the Assessment and Treatment of Depression, Anxiety, and Substance Use Disorders

Jane E. Fisher, Michael A. Cucciare, Claudia Droßel, and Craig Yury

DEPRESSION IN OLDER ADULTS

Basic Facts About Depression

The term *depression* refers to a wide variety of mood presentations, with the most severely debilitating being *major depression*. According to the *Diagnostic and Statistical Manual of Mental Disorders*, Fourth Edition (*DSM—IV*; American Psychiatric Association, 1994), major depression is characterized by the presence of five or more of the following symptoms occurring during the same two-week period accompanied by a change in previous functioning: depressed mood every (or nearly every) day; loss of interest in pleasurable activities; changes in weight (not due to dieting) in a month period; problems sleeping (or oversleeping) nearly every day; psychomotor agitation, fatigue or loss of energy; feelings of worthlessness and guilt; difficulties concentrating and making decisions; and thoughts of death or suicide. As part of the diagnostic criteria for major depression, these symptoms must cause (a) clinically significant distress or impairment in occupational, social, or other important areas of functioning; (b) not be the result of medication or a medical condition; and (c) not occur due to bereavement.

Depression is the most common psychiatric disorder among the elderly (Zauszniewski, Morris, Preechawong, & Chang, 2004), with prevalence ranging from 1% in healthy individuals to 50% in individuals with medical illness (Mittman et al., 1997). Women are twice as likely as males to experience depression (Garber & Flynn, 2001). Comorbid psychological problems include anxiety, substance use and eating disorders; borderline and histrionic personality disorders; and somatization (i.e., physical complaints such as headaches and back pain) (Stefanis & Stefanis, 1999). Common comorbid medical conditions include dementia, Alzheimer's disease, diabetes, Parkinson's disease, stroke, cardiovascular disease, cancer, and HIV/AIDS.

The most serious complication of depression is suicide (American Psychiatric Association, 1994); as many as 55% of suicidal older adults suffer from depression (Draper, 1996). Furthermore, suicide rates are highest among adults age 65 and older; although this age group makes up only 13% of the U.S. population, its members account for 20% of all suicide deaths (United Sates Department of Health and Human Services, 1999).

Assessment of Depressive Disorders

What Should Be Ruled Out?

When assessing depression, one should rule out a major depressive episode due to coexisting medical conditions or substance use disorders; and general medical conditions that can produce a major depressive episode (e.g., diabetes, hypothyroidism, brain tumors, anemia, and metabolic abnormalities). A physician should be consulted when a medical condition is thought to be contributing to the presence of a major depressive episode.

What Is Involved in Effective Assessment?

A thorough assessment of depression should include screening for symptoms of depression, severity of depressive symptoms, suicidal ideation/past attempts, presence of psychotic symptoms, history of manic episode, history of recurrent depression, substance use, medical history (e.g., date of last physical exam), functional disabilities (e.g., missed work days), life stressors, family and other forms of social support/social isolation, and involvement in activities.

Assessment Instruments for Screening and Diagnosing Depression in Older Adults

Table 5.1 summarizes seven evidence-based assessment instruments, based on sound psychometric data, for assessing symptom severity and/or diagnosing depression in older adults. These evidence-based instruments are used (a) in specific settings, (b) with specific populations (e.g., medically ill or

TABLE 5.1   Evidence-Based Instruments for Assessing Symptoms of Depression in Older Adults

Instrument	Specific Settings	Specific Populations	Specific Purposes	Other Findings
The Center for Epidemiological Studies Depression Scale (CES-D) (Radloff, 1977) 20-item CES-D 8-item CES-D (Mojtabai & Olfson, 2004)	Assess depressive symptoms in medical and nonmedical samples of older adults (Sawyer-Radloff & Teri, 1986). Use its 8-item form in fast-paced medical settings such as primary clinics (Mojtabai & Olfson, 2004).	Used in ethnically diverse populations (Liang, Tran, Krause, & Markides, 1989). The 8-item form is used in older adults experiencing cognitive deficits (or possible dementia) (Mojtabai & Olfson, 2004).	Both planning treatment and monitoring treatment outcomes in depressed, multiethnic populations of older adults (Coon, Thompson, Steffen, Sorocco, & Gallagher-Thompson, 2003; Gallagher et al., 2003).	CES-D performed poorly in detecting both minor and major depression in adults age 75 and older (Watson, Lewis, Kistler, Amick, & Boustani, 2004).
The Geriatric Depression Scale (GDS) 5-items; Sheikh & Yesavage, 1986)	Assess symptom severity in depressed older adults in medical settings (Sood, Cisek, Zimmerman, Zaleski, & Filmore, 2003).	In older adults with histories of trauma (Cook, Areán, Schnurr, Sheikh, 2001). In older adults with comorbid mental health problems such as schizophrenia (Graham, Arthur, & Howard, 2002).	To track treatment outcomes (Scogin, 1987) and to use for treatment planning and monitoring treatment outcomes (Sood et al., 2003).	GDS may not be the most effective assessment for identifying depression in adults age 75 and older (Watson et al., 2004).

(continue)

TABLE 5.1   Evidence-Based Instruments for Assessing Symptoms of Depression in Older Adults

Instrument	Specific Settings	Specific Populations	Specific Purposes	Other Findings
Hamilton Depression Rating Scale (HAM-D) 23-item form (Hamilton, 1960) 17-item form, an extracted-HDRS (Rapp, Smith, & Britt, 1990).	In medical settings (Cook, Areán, Schnurr, Sheikh, 2001).	In depressed older adults experiencing memory difficulties (Harwood, Barker, Ownby, Mullan, & Duara, 2004). In older adults with histories of trauma (Cook, Areán, Schnurr, Sheikh, 2001).	Assess symptom severity and track treatment outcomes (Sirey, Bruce, & Alexopoulos, 2005). HDRS scores are associated with emotional expressivity in depressed older adults (Wagner, Logsdon, Pearson, & Teri, 1997).	The concurrent validity of the Extracted-HDRS is well established using the GDS and the BDI (Rapp, Smith, & Britt, 1990.)
Beck Depression Inventory-II (BDI-II) 21 items (Beck, Steer, & Brown, 1996)	In medical and nonmedical settings (Goldberg, Breckenridge, & Sheikh, 2003; Ashendorf, Constantinou, & McCaffrey, 2004).	In older adults with memory difficulties (Williams, Little, Scates, & Blockman, 1987).	To track treatment outcomes in depressed older adults (Hamblin, Beutler, Scogin, & Corbishley, 1993).	None

Structured Clinical Interview for DSM-IV Axis I (SCID—I) (First, Spitzer, Gibbon, & Williams, 1996, 1997)	In medical settings (Williams, Little, Scates, & Blockman, 1987).	In older adults with memory difficulties (Williams et al., 1987). In frail, older adults (Wagner, Logsdon, Pearson, & Teri, 1997).	None	None
Diagnostic Interview Schedule—IV (DIS—IV) (Robins, Helzer, Croughan, & Ratcliff, 1981)	In medical settings (Areán & Alvidrez, 2001).	In a community-based sample of older adults (Beekman, Deeg, Van Limbeek, & Braam, 1997). In medically ill, low-income older adults (Areán & Alvidrez, 2001).	None	The DIS-IV has good criterion validity with regard to diagnosing depression when compared to the CES-D (Beekman et al., 1997).
Primary Care Evaluations of Mental Disorders (PRIME-MD) (Spitzer et al., 1995)	In home care settings (Preville, Cote, Boyer, & Hebert, 2004).	In frail, older adults receiving home healthcare services (Preville et al., 2004).	None	May be limited in discriminating among older adults (Preville et al., 2004).

low-income), and (c) for specific purposes (e.g., monitoring treatment outcomes and treatment planning).

Evidence-Based Intervention for Depression

What Is Effective Medical Treatment?

The best evidence supports the use of tricyclic antidepressants (TCAs), selective serotonin reuptake inhibitors (SSRIs), serotonin/norepinephrine reuptake inhibitors (SNRIs), monoamine oxidase inhibitors (MAOIs), and antidepressants such as buproprian and trazadone for the treatment of depression (Howard & Bandyopadhyay, 1993; Mittman et al., 1997). These medications appear to be equally effective (Padala, Roccaforte, & Burke, 2004) in their short-term effects, although it is unclear how these medications should be used to prevent relapse.

Treatment guidelines for antidepressant use among older adults have generally been derived from research on the general population. However, research on the use of antidepressants in older adults (e.g., Howard & Bandyopadhyay, 1993; see Mittman et al., 1997, for a meta-analysis) generally concludes/recommends that older adults have similar rates of unwanted side effects regardless of the type of antidepressant taken (i.e., TCAs, SSRIs, and MAOIs); no antidepressant class is superior with respect to efficacy for treating depression in older adults; there is little advantage to prescribing one class of antidepressant over another when treating depression in older adults; there is little known about the long-term efficacy of antidepressants in older adults; ideal antidepressants for use by an older adults should be efficacious, free of or have limited unwanted side effects, safe in overdose, have a predictable metabolism, and be safe in combination with other psychotropic medication; and an ideal antidepressant for the aged would be given once per day at a fixed dose.

What Are Effective Therapist-Based Treatments?

Cognitive behavioral therapy (CBT), behavior therapy (BT), and interpersonal therapy (IPT) are each effective in the treatment of depression for older adults. This section presents information on common components and length of treatment for each therapy model.

Cognitive Behavioral Therapy. CBT characterizes depression as a consequence of dysfunctional patterns of thinking and low rates of pleasurable experiences. The underlying theory is that by changing maladaptive patterns of thinking and increasing involvement in pleasurable activities, clients will experience a subsequent change in affect and behavior (Beck, Rush, Shaw, & Emery, 1979). CBT consists of several components, including teaching clients (a) to understand the link between thinking and behaving, and feelings of depression; (b) to identify and better cope with unhelpful thinking patterns; (c) to monitor daily mood and frequency of engaging in pleasant events; (d) to identify obstacles to engaging in pleasant activities; (e) goal setting; (f) contingency management (i.e., learning how to reward oneself for achieving goals); (g) problem-solving skills; and (h) relaxation training (see Beck et al., 1979; Free, 1999 for CBT with nonelderly populations; see Gallagher-Thompson et al., 2000; Gallagher-Thompson et al., 2003; Coon, Thompson, Steffen, Sorocco, & Gallagher-Thompson, 2003 for CBT with older adults). A typical course of treatment ranges from 10 to 16 weekly sessions.

Behavior Therapy. BT defines depression as a consequence of decreased access to reinforcing experiences. The focus of BT is to increase clients' access to reinforcing activities with the purpose of elevating mood (Martell, Addis, & Jacobson, 2001). The most notable treatment component of BT for treating depression is behavioral activation (BA). BA teaches clients that they become depressed when they stop behaving in a goal directed manner, and it therefore promotes goal-directed behavior in depressed patients. BA uses (a) a functional assessment to identify environmental triggers for the depression and clients' responses (e.g., avoidance) to those triggers; (b) relaxation and social skills training; (c) focused activation to help clients engage in goal-directed activities; (d) graded task assignment (i.e., the process by which clients engage in more difficult tasks and completion of a goal); and (e) self-monitoring to track mood and the patient's behavior from day to day (see Martell et al., 2001, for an overview of behavioral activation theory and techniques; see Masters, Burish, Hollon, & Rimm, 1987, for an overview of behavior therapy; see Coon et al., 2003, for group treatment for older adults). A typical course of treatment ranges from 10 to 12 weekly sessions.

Interpersonal Therapy. IPT posits that depression is caused, made worse, or maintained by interpersonal difficulties. Therefore, IPT therapists focus on resolving interpersonal difficulties to alleviate depression (Areán, 2004). IPT therapists first educate clients about depression and the factors (i.e., interpersonal difficulties) that contribute to their mood. Following education, IPT therapists attempt to identify the interpersonal difficulties that contribute most to a client's mood. The four most common areas of interpersonal conflict are unresolved grief, role transitions, interpersonal role disputes, and interpersonal deficits. Clients are then taught to identify the relationship between their interpersonal difficulties and mood. Homework is assigned throughout treatment to help clients overcome or cope with their interpersonal difficulties (see Areán, 2004, for brief overview of IPT). A typical course of treatment ranges from 16 to 28 weekly sessions.

What Is Effective Self-Help Treatment?

There are several self-help books that contain information on the preceding treatments. Three of the most popular self-help books providing information on evidence-based treatment of depression are *Feeling Good: The New Mood Therapy* (2nd ed.), by D. D. Burns (1999a); *The Feeling Good Handbook*, by D. D. Burns (1999b); and *Control Your Depression*, by P. M. Lewinsohn, R. F. Munoz, M. A. Youngren, and A. M. Zeiss (1992).

Useful Web sites include:

- American Psychological Association at http://www.apa.org/topics/topic_depress.html
- Depression.com at http://www.depression.com
- WebMD Depression Health Center at http://my.webmd.com/medical_information/condition_centers/depression/default.htm
- National Institute of Mental Health at http://www.nimh.nih.gov/health information/depressionmenu.cfm

Other Issues in the Treatment and Management of Depression

A positive response to psychotherapy is typically seen between 8 and 12 weeks, and a positive response to medications is usually seen before 6 weeks. Patients who respond to antidepressant medications should continue to receive the full therapeutic dose of medications for at least 6 months following symptomatic recovery; if the patient does not show signs of improvement within 4 to 6 weeks, modification of medical dosage or intervention should occur. There is some evidence that demonstrates the superiority of both medication and psychotherapy in treating older adults with depression (Dew et al., 2001). However, these findings show that response to depression treatment (i.e., medication alone, psychotherapy alone, or combined medication and psychotherapy) can depend on individuals' response to treatment within the first 16 weeks. For example, individuals who demonstrated at least some change in depressive symptoms during this time were more likely to display reduced symptoms of depression during the maintenance phase when receiving combined treatment.

How Does One Select Among Treatments?

There are few studies that examine methods for choosing among possible treatments for depression in older adults (Dew et al., 2001; Unutzer et al., 2003). Findings from Dew et al. suggest that individuals who display rapid initial responses to treatment do well receiving either medication or psychotherapy, while individuals who show mixed (or slower) initial responses to treatment may do better in the long term when receiving combined treatment for depression. In addition to the initial response to treatment, there are a variety of other factors that may be considered when deciding among treatments.

- *Assess possible side effects of medication, differential compliance to various treatment modalities, and patient preference.* Persons taking medication to treat depression may experience a wide variety of side effects (Mittman et al., 1997), which may reduce their willingness to adhere to treatment. Older adults have the highest rates of medication nonadherence than any other age group, and depression can further interfere with adherence to medication use (Erickson & Muramatsu, 2004). In addition, after examining treatment preferences of approximately 1,800 depressed older adults, Unutzer et al. (2003) found that the majority of individuals preferred psychotherapy over medication for treating depression; however, the exact reasons for this preference are not clearly understood. Thus, when choosing among possible treatment options it is important for the provider to assess possible barriers (e.g., side effects and depressive symptoms) to treatment adherence and specific factors (e.g., availability of time, beliefs about treatment options) that can contribute to patient preferences.
- *Examine previous response to treatment(s).* The findings from the Dew et al. (2001) study suggest that previous and initial response to treatment may play an important role in predicting which treatments will be most effective in the long term. Regarding medication therapy, Rothschild (1996) points out that there are several classes of medication that can be used to effectively treat depression in older adults. Therefore if one class of medication is found to be ineffective, a medication from another class should be prescribed.
- *Consider the physical health and medical conditions that can cause and contribute to feelings of depression.* Many of these factors (e.g., diabetes) can be managed medically. Medical comorbidity can play a role in choosing among types of treatments. For example, Padala et al. (2004) point out that TCAs should be used with caution in individuals with cardiac disease due to increased risk of heart rate, orthostatic hypotension, and

prolonged cardiac conduction. Also, TCAs should not be used with individuals with dementia, narrow-angle glaucoma, urinary retention, or bowel obstruction due to the anticholinergic properties of this class of medication (see Padala et al., 2004, for a more thorough discussion of selection criteria). Thus, individuals presenting with medical problems should be seen by a physician to rule out medical conditions before treatment is decided on.

ANXIETY IN OLDER ADULTS

Basic Facts About Anxiety

The *Diagnostic and Statistical Manual of Mental Disorders*, Fourth Edition (*DSM—IV—TR*; American Psychiatric Association, 2000), defines anxiety as "the apprehensive anticipation of future danger or misfortune accompanied by a feeling of dysphoria or somatic symptoms of tension" (p. 820). All anxiety disorders share cognitive (e.g., worry) and physiological (e.g., tension or arousal) characteristics. Their topographically dissimilar behavioral patterns serve the same consequence, namely, avoidance of or escape from anxiety-producing events or situations. As the *DSM—IV—TR* (2000) notes, these events or situations can be external (e.g., lightning) or internal (e.g., somatic sensations, cognitions) and their avoidance must interfere significantly with daily functioning. See Table 5.2 for a brief overview of the anxiety disorders.

Although anxiety disorders were once considered rare in older adults, critical analyses revealed methodological problems and suggested a gross underestimation of anxiety. In addition, Fuentes and Cox (1997) reasoned that prevalence data regarding anxiety disorders in the elderly might be skewed toward underestimation due to the high prevalence of comorbid conditions: anxious behavior tends to co-occur with depressive behavior and with medical conditions; the tendency of older adults to complain about somatic ailments that do not meet *DSM—IV* diagnostic criteria (e.g., trembling, muscle tension or aches, restlessness, easy fatigability, tightness around the head, lump in throat, autonomic hyperactivity, shortness of breath, palpitations, sweating, dry mouth, dizziness, nausea, frequent urination, edginess, exaggerated startle response, difficulty concentrating, trouble falling or staying asleep, and irritability (Salzman & Sheikh, 2005); and the tendency of elderly with medical conditions to be bound to the home. Current prevalence estimates of anxiety in the elderly are as high as 20% (with diagnosable anxiety between 5% and 10%), making anxiety disorders more common than major depression, dysthymia, or severe cognitive impairment among people

TABLE 5.2   Anxiety Disorders

Disorder	Panic attacks necessary for diagnosis?	Avoidance of or escape from . . .	Worry about . . .	Duration of worry and avoidance
Panic disorder without agoraphobia	Yes (recurrent and unexpected)	Somatic sensations	Panic attacks and their consequences, particularly physical threat	At least 1 month
with agoraphobia	Yes (recurrent and unexpected)	Somatic sensations and places	Being unable to escape or to receive help when having a panic attack	At least 1 month
Specific phobia	No	Specific events, animals, and objects	Specific events, animals, and objects	
Social phobia	No	Social and performance situations	Being scrutinized, embarrassed, or having negative social impact	
Obsessive-compulsive disorder	No	Persistent cognitions, e.g., ideas, thoughts, impulses, images	e.g., contamination, destruction or loss of property	
Posttraumatic stress disorder	No	Reminders of traumatic event	Reexperiencing/recurrence of the traumatic event	At least 1 month
Acute stress disorder	No	Reminders of traumatic event	Reexperiencing/recurrence of the traumatic event	Within 4 weeks after traumatic event
Generalized anxiety disorder	No (rare)	Worry and, more generally, negative affective states	Routine life circumstances: health, family, finances, work	At least 6 months

over the age of 65 (Wetherell, 1998). Moreover, de Beurs et al. (1999) found that elderly whose reported anxiety did not meet criteria for diagnosis experienced the same effects of anxiety on physical and psychological well-being as those elderly who had been diagnosed.

Anxiety disorders have been correlated with a decline in cardiovascular health and increased mortality; incidence of hypertension; high cholesterol levels and risk of coronary artery disease; excess use of health services; decrease in quality of life; and compromised psychosocial functioning (for a review, see Alwahhabi, 2003). Additionally, anxiety has been found to be a significant predictor of pain in older adults (Feeney, 2004).

Assessment of Anxiety Disorders

What Must Be Ruled Out?

For effective treatment planning, primary anxiety disorders must be distinguished from anxiety disorders due to a general medical condition and substance-induced anxiety disorders. The specification of a medical condition is indicated when an anxiety disorder is a direct result of medical pathology, such as endocrine, cardiovascular, respiratory, metabolic, and neurological conditions (*DSM—IV—TR*; American Psychiatric Association, 2000, p. 478).

Practitioners are alerted to the possibility of substance-induced anxiety disorder if anxiety, panic, or obsessions and compulsions have developed within one month of substance use or withdrawal. Intoxication from a variety of substances, for example, alcohol or caffeine, is associated with anxiety disorders as is withdrawal from many substances, such as alcohol, sedatives, hypnotics, or anxiolytics. The *DSM—IV—TR* also specifies classes of medications that might prompt anxiety, such as analgesics, sympathomimetics or other bronchodilators, anticholinergics, insulin, thyroid preparations, antihistamines, cardiovascular medications, and antipsychotic and antidepressant medications.

When a primary anxiety disorder cannot be clearly differentiated from anxiety disorder due to a medical condition or substance-induced anxiety disorder, then the anxiety disorder receives the label, "not otherwise specified." This label also applies when avoidance patterns significantly interrupt daily functioning, yet not all diagnostic criteria are met; when neither depression nor an anxiety disorder can be pinpointed ("mixed anxiety-depressive disorder"); and when the social impact of a diagnosed medical or behavioral problem occasions clinically significant avoidance of social situations.

Assessment Instruments for Evaluating Anxiety Disorders in Older Adults

The psychometric properties of most measures of anxiety apply to the assessment of younger adults. Following their evaluation with older adults, the following measures are recommended or interpreted as holding promise for the use with older populations by Beck and Stanley (2001): *Clinician-rated measures: Anxiety Disorders Interview Schedule* (Brown, DiNardo, & Barlow, 1994), *Structured Clinical Interview for DSM—IV* (First, Spitzer, Gibbon, & Williams, 1996); and *Hamilton Anxiety Rating Scale* (Hamilton, 1959) see Table 5.3.

The psychometric properties of specific assessments for acute and chronic posttraumatic stress disorder (PTSD) have not been determined for community samples of older adults (Busuttil, 2004). Measures evaluated with younger adults or specific elderly populations (e.g., treatment-seeking

TABLE 5.3   Instruments for Assessing Anxiety Symptoms

Instrument	Length (items)	Specific Purposes
Beck Anxiety Inventory (A. T. Beck & Steer, 1993)	21	Designed to discriminate anxiety from depression (See Wetherell & Gatz, 2005).
Fear Questionnaire subscales (Marks & Matthews, 1979; Stanley, Novy, Bourland, Beck, & Averill, 2001)	15	Assesses for specific phobias.
Hopkins Symptom Checklist (Derogatis, Lipman, Rickels, Uhlenhuth, & Covi, 1974)	58	Comprising five factors assessing somatization, obsessive-compulsive, interpersonal sensitivity, depression, and anxiety.
Padua Inventory (Sanavio, 1988)	60	Assess obsessions and compulsions.
Penn State Worry Questionnaire (Meyer, Miller, Metzger, & Borkovec, 1990)	16	Assess excessive and uncontrollable worry and to discriminate generalized anxiety disorder from other anxiety disorders.
State-Trait Anxiety Inventory (Spielberger, Gorsuch, Lushene, Vagg, & Jacobs, 1983)	20	Designed to detect trait anxiety.
Worry Scale (Wisocki, Handen, & Morse, 1986)	35	Designed to assess specific content areas of worry.
Zung Self-Rating Anxiety Scale (Zung, 1971)	20	Assess primarily somatic complaints (15 out of 20 items).

veterans, Holocaust survivors) include: *Clinician-Administered PTSD Scale* (CAPS; Blake et al., 1990; 1995; see also Weathers, Ruscio, & Keane, 1999); *Posttraumatic Diagnostic Scale* (Foa, Cashman, Jaycox, & Perry, 1997) with 49 items, follows the *DSM—IV* criteria for PTSD; *Trauma Symptom Inventory* (Briere, 1995; Briere, Elliot, Harris, & Cotman, 1995) with 100 items, follows the *DSM—IV* criteria for PTSD and is also designed to assess interpersonal problems as well as underreporting, overreporting, and inconsistent response style.

For an extensive review of psychometric properties of measures for acute and posttraumatic stress disorder, see Orsillo, Batten, and Hammond (2001). As a general strategy, Busuttil (2004) recommends multimodal assessment. The combined use of self-report scales, clinical interviews, and behavioral assessments, such as anxiety ratings (Wolpe & Lazarus, 1966) or self-monitoring, should render information about the key features or properties of the anxiety-related problem, development and course of the problem, degree of interference with daily functioning (e.g., intensity, frequency), comorbidity, treatment history and preferences, personal history (e.g., life changes due to retirement, bereavement), medical history, family history, and possible skills deficits that might contribute to anxiety (Antony, 2001, p. 13). Kogan, Edelstein, and McKee (2000) provide a detailed review and recommendations for the assessment of older adults.

Special Considerations in the Assessment of Anxiety in Older Adults

Assessment of anxiety in older adults warrants the following special considerations (see Beck & Stanley, 2001; Kane, 2000, pp. 11–12):

- *Has effective communication with the older adult been established?* Does auditory decline make it necessary to face the respondent and to carefully enunciate each word? Has background noise been eliminated? Does visual decline require additional lighting? Are written materials printed with larger font (preferably Arial 14)?
- *Are the sessions scheduled at an appropriate time?* Have transportation barriers (e.g., heavy traffic, difficulties with way-finding) been discussed? Has the client's risk of fatigue (e.g., due to a medical condition) been assessed and has session duration been adjusted accordingly?
- *Could medical and medication issues interfere with assessment?* Has cognitive impairment been considered?
- *Is sufficient time provided?* Is the interviewer prepared to patiently wait for answers to questions or to provide reminders or prompts, as necessary? Can the interviewer accommodate inappropriate answers that

might be a function of social deprivation? Would it be helpful to provide the client with a list of questions to prepare for the next assessment session?

- *Does the interviewer's style facilitate accurate reporting?* Is the use of less professional jargon (e.g., "distress") and more concrete terms indicated? Given the potentially large age discrepancy between therapist and client, is the therapist prepared to ask questions that might be embarrassing to both therapist and client? Is it necessary to obtain a release to corroborate information with other individuals?

Evidence-Based Interventions for Anxiety

What Are Effective Drug Treatments?

Wetherell's (1998) review of available treatments for anxiety in older adults notes that "most older adults who receive treatment for anxiety are treated with medications" (p. 445). Accordingly, four anxiolytics of the benzodiazepine class—alprazolam, clonazepam, diazepam, and lorazepam—have been among the 100 most commonly prescribed medications (Longo & Johnson, 2000), although their long-term use is associated with a higher risk of injury (Tamblyn, Abrahamowicz, du Berger, McLeod, & Bartlett, 2005) and with an increase in the rate of postoperative confusion (Kudoh, Takase, Takahira, & Takazawa, 2004). Most important, long-term use of benzodiazepines also constitutes a risk factor for cognitive decline and dementia (Paterniti, Dufouil, & Alperovitch, 2002; Stewart, 2005; Verdoux, Lagnaoui, & Begaud, 2005; for a general review of drug-induced cognitive impairments in the elderly, see Gray, Lai, & Larson, 1999). Additional adverse effects include sedation, psychomotor impairment, respiratory depression, urinary incontinence, and substance dependence (Salzman, 2005). For this reason, even short-term benzodiazepine administration should be weighed with caution and its use tapered off gradually (Sheikh, 2004).

Nonbenzodiazepine drug interventions for anxiety disorders include the administration of antidepressants, buspirone, beta-blockers, antihistamines, and neuroleptics (for a review of the literature, see Salzman, 2005). As Salzman (2005, p. 467) points out, "the more severe the [anxiety] disorder, the lower the likelihood of response to medication." The upward-titration of dosages to reach the desired therapeutic effect correlates with an increased risk in adverse and potentially irreversible drug effects (e.g., tardive dyskinesia), particularly when the older adult is taking multiple medications. Paradoxically, because of dose-dependent and idiosyncratic effects, the administration of these nonbenzodiazepine drugs has also been linked to an increase in anxiety (see the preceding discussion of substance-induced anxiety). Salzman (2005) points out that no empirical studies for using these drugs with older patients are available. Consequently, in principle each drug prescription, titration, or withdrawal would warrant a careful monitoring of the potential therapeutic and adverse effects according to single-subject experimentation guidelines (Kollins, Ehrhardt, & Poling, 2000).

What Are Effective Therapist-Based Treatments?

As described earlier, anxiety disorders share cognitive and physiological characteristics, and they involve avoidance of or escape from anxiety-producing events or situations. Accordingly, evidence-based interventions for anxiety disorders typically employ three major components, in isolation or in any combination: (1) an intervention focusing on cognitive changes, (2) relaxation techniques, and (3) graduated exposure to feared events or situations.

Cognitive Component. Cognitive changes are brought about by cognitive restructuring (Dobson & Hamilton, 2003; Ellis, 2003; Newman, 2003), or cognitive defusion (Luoma & Hayes, 2003). Both techniques address the verbal barriers (reasons, rules, logic) that might accompany the avoidance of events. While restructuring techniques focus on providing the client with new rules (e.g., by training thought-stopping, coping self-statements, alternative thoughts, and logical errors), defusion techniques teach the client to notice the self-talk (reason giving, blaming, evaluating) as a correlate of behavior without a necessarily causal role. Defusion thus aims at changing the impact of thoughts on behavior in general by emphasizing that, regardless of the nature of accompanying thoughts, any action can be chosen. Restructuring does not question the relationship of thoughts and behavior in principle, but supplies new—more functional—reasons, rules, or logic. In addition to cognitive restructuring or cognitive defusion, the treatment package might also include a skill-building component (e.g., problem-solving skills, interpersonal skills).

Relaxation Techniques. Relaxation techniques include behavioral relaxation training (Ferguson, 2003), diaphragmatic breathing (Hazlett-Stevens & Craske, 2003), or forms of yoga and meditation. All relaxation techniques teach the recognition of increased autonomic arousal or tension and target a decrease. A study by Scogin, Rickard, Keith, Wilson, and McElreath (1992) illustrates the effectiveness of progressive and imaginal relaxation training for elderly persons with subjective anxiety.

Exposure. Exposure techniques involve the confrontation of previously avoided events or situations. This confrontation might occur in vivo or it might be imagined. Imagined exposure is recommended as a first step when clients are reluctant to enter actual situations or if the actual situation cannot be generated. Importantly, exposure exercises are always designed to produce distress that is acceptable to the client. The duration of exposure is contingent on a reported substantial reduction of peak anxiety levels within a session.

The selection of specific exposure techniques depends on the nature of the avoided event and also takes into account the topography and the severity of the avoidant behavior patterns (e.g., if contamination is avoided through cleaning rituals, the effective prevention of these rituals constitutes part of the exposure treatment). Medication with anxiolytic properties might diminish the effects of exposure-based interventions (e.g., Spiegel & Bruce, 1997).

- *Panic disorder.* By holding their breath, breathing through a straw, climbing stairs, spinning, hyperventilating, or rebreathing expired air, clients generate cardiopulmonary conditions that have a high probability of producing panic and avoidance behavior. Such interceptive exposure is very effective and can be applied in individual or group therapy sessions (Forsyth & Fusé, 2003); however, it is contraindicated when cardiopulmonary or cardiovascular diseases are present. Forsyth and Fusé (2003) provide a brief review and detailed instructions on the selection and implementation of interceptive exposure; see also Craske and Barlow (2001). Swales, Solfvin, and Sheikh (1996) used interceptive exposure as part of a larger cognitive-behavioral therapy (CBT) package with 15 older adults and found it effective. Garfinkel (1979) and Rathus and Sanderson (1996) provide additional case reports of significant improvement after implementing CBT for panic disorder with older adults.
- *Specific phobias.* Gradual exposure-based interventions require clients, in collaboration with the therapist, to establish a hierarchy of avoided objects, animals, or events for gradual exposure starting with the least feared item. Hazlett-Stevens and Craske (2003) provide a brief overview and a step-by-step approach to gradual in vivo exposure; see Head and Gross (2003) for details on arranging imagined exposure sessions. Significant improvement may occur after only a single intensive exposure session; the plethora of data on the effectiveness and efficacy of exposure for specific phobias has made it the first-line intervention (e.g., Öst,

1989). Fabian and Haley (1991), Thyer (1981), and Wanderer (1972) provide case reports on exposure-based interventions for specific phobias with older adults.

- *Social phobia.* As in other exposure-based interventions for specific phobias, clients construct a fear hierarchy. Generating an anxiety-provoking social context and managing social interactions within it constitutes the exposure session. Social skill training is usually included within the treatment package. For a detailed review and a step-by-step approach to implementation, see Turk, Heimberg, and Hope (2001). The application of available and efficacious exposure-based treatments for social phobia with elder adults has not yet been studied, although Sheikh and Cassidy (2000) suggest that elderly people who tend to avoid writing or eating in public (e.g., as a function of tremors or dental problems) might benefit.

- *Obsessive compulsive disorder.* Evidence-based interventions for obsessive-compulsive disorder consist of exposure to events that evoke obsessions while voluntarily refraining from engaging in ritualized avoidance behaviors (e.g., hand washing, checking). Here, too, gradual exposure is preferable to maintain the client's motivation by providing opportunities for success (i.e., report of decreased anxiety levels) within a session. Calamari, Faber, Hitsman, and Poppe (1994); Junginger and Ditto (1984); Rowan, Holburn, Walker, and Siddiqui (1984); and Turner, Hersen, Bellack, and Wells (1979) provide case examples involving application of the techniques with older adults.

- *Posttraumatic stress disorder.* The exposure component for PTSD involves reliving the traumatic event through imagined means and experiencing in vivo fear-producing situations related to the event. The *Practice Guidelines from the International Society for Traumatic Stress Studies* (Foa, Keane, & Friedman, 2000) concluded that the use of exposure therapy was well supported (Rothbaum, Meadows, Resick, & Foy, 2000). Because chronic PTSD frequently occurs with other behavioral problems, recent treatment packages have taken a broad-spectrum approach. They address comorbidity in the form of substance use or other affective disorders (Lombardo & Gray, 2005). Treatments that have demonstrated usefulness with younger adults have not been systematically studied with community-sampled older adults (but for an application of exposure therapy using virtual reality with combat veterans, see Rothbaum, Hodges, Ready, Graap, and Alarcon, 2001).

- *Generalized anxiety disorder.* Individuals with generalized anxiety disorder tend to worry about negative affective states (e.g., Ruscio &

Borkovec, 2004). Thus, while exposure techniques for generalized anxiety disorder used to focus on tolerating worrisome situations (e.g., being late), the current approach also emphasizes exposure to worrying in particular and negative affective states, in general. For a step-by-step approach, see Brown, O'Leary, and Barlow (2001). Cognitive-behavioral therapy is an effective treatment for generalized anxiety disorder in younger adults and has been studied with older adults (see Stanley & Novy, 2000). Mohlman (2004) reviewed the available literature on the use of treatment packages involving exposure and concluded that "non-standard and augmented therapies (e.g., CBT with a medical aspect, with learning aids, or delivered in patients' own homes) appear to produce best results" (p. 164). This flexible and individualized approach, based on the person's educational and skill level, is also showing promise for the scores of older adults with anxiety and concurrent medical problems or cognitive impairment, who were not believed to benefit from nonpharmacological interventions (Mohlman, 2004).

Overall Efficacy

Although the efficacy of these interventions with older adults has been chronically understudied, Nordhus and Pallesen (2003) provided a meta-analysis of 15 outcome studies involving participants who were 63 to 84 years of age and reported anxiety or had diagnoses of panic disorder with and without agoraphobia, social phobia, generalized anxiety disorder, and anxiety disorder not otherwise specified. The investigators found that the meta-analysis of interventions based on the preceding conceptualizations demonstrated "significant improvements in self-reported, as well as diagnosed, anxiety in older adults at post-treatment" (p. 648). Combinations of cognitive behavioral strategies for the treatment of PTSD have demonstrated effectiveness in the younger adult literature (for a review, see Herbert & Forman, in press), but they have not been systematically studied with older adults (Averill & Beck, 2000; Weintraub & Ruskin, 1999).

Modifications of Treatment Components

The modifications of treatment protocols for younger adults have not been systematized for older adults, but the following modifications can be found/ suggested in the literature: increase overall duration of treatment, decrease session length, increase effort to accommodate clients when scheduling (e.g., including home visits and telephone calls), simplification of treatment procedures, homework forms and terminology, use of mnemonic aids, use of multiple modalities for teaching, pacing skill-building components according to the client's progress, and involving family members in skill-building components.

SUBSTANCE USE DISORDERS IN OLDER ADULTS

Basic Facts About Substance Abuse

Substance abuse in older adults is associated with poor health prognosis, increased disability, high health-care utilization, increased mortality, and higher suicide rate (Bartels, Blow, Brockman, & Van Citters, 2005).

The *DSM* criteria for substance abuse may not be appropriate for older adults as age-associated changes in physiology and pharmokinetics can alter the presentation of tolerance and dependence (Patterson, Lacro, & Jeste, 1999). Compared to younger adults, the development of tolerance in an older adult may involve minimal or no increase in the consumption of alcohol necessary to produce intoxication due to changes in physiology (e.g., a slower metabolic rate). Therefore, *DSM* criteria for tolerance and dependence may be invalid indicators of substance abuse in older adults.

The majority of older adults who abuse alcohol began drinking at a younger age and continued the pattern into late life. Approximately, one-third of older alcoholic patients started drinking as older adults (American Medical Association, 1996). Many persons with early-onset alcoholism survive to develop alcohol-related illnesses compounded by changes associated with aging. Research has demonstrated that earlier onset of substance abuse is related to greater risk for substance dependence and poorer treatment outcomes (SAMSHA, 2002).

Gender differences in clinical characteristics, treatment retention, and outcome of alcohol-dependent older adults have not been fully investigated. It has been suggested that women are more likely than men to start drinking heavily later in life (Menninger, 2002). Overall, men appear more likely to abuse alcohol: Studies have shown that 15% of elderly men and 12% of elderly women regularly drank in excess of one standard drink per day (Adams, Barry, & Fleming, 1996), while 13% of elderly men and 2% of elderly women are heavy users (Mirand & Welte, 1996). Older women are prescribed more and consume more psychoactive drugs, particularly benzodiazepines, than are men and are more likely to be long-term users of these substances (Gomberg, 1995).

Alcohol and Illegal Substances

The prevalence of alcohol consumption in elderly populations as well as the associated risk of abuse is illustrated by the following statistics:

- 45% of community-dwelling adults over age 50 consume alcohol (SAMSHA, 2005).
- 6% to 16% of older adults are considered heavy users (i.e., more than two drinks per day; Mirand & Welte, 1996).
- 7.2% of adults over age 65 report binge alcohol use and 1.8% report heavy drinking (SAMSHA, 2005).
- 49% of institutionalized populations met criteria for lifetime alcohol abuse or dependence, 18% met criteria for current alcohol abuse or dependence (Joseph, Ganzini, & Atkinson, 1995)

Patients with late-onset alcoholism as compared to early onset have greater resources and family support, and are more likely to complete treatment and to have somewhat better outcomes (Liberto & Oslin, 1995; Schutte, Brennan, & Moos, 1994). These findings are associated with the consequences of limited financial and social resources experienced by persons with a history of chronic substance abuse.

Physiological Correlates of Chronic Alcohol Abuse

Cognitive Impairment. Long-term abuse of alcohol can lead to neurological dysfunction (Kril, Halliday, Svoboda, & Cartwright, 1997). Global cognitive impairment is most common, resulting in an alcohol-related dementia that may be accompanied by profound cerebral atrophy.

- Frontal lobe dysfunction is most frequently encountered in alcoholics.
- Excluding Alzheimer's disease, rates of all types of dementia are higher in people with alcohol abuse (Thomas & Rockwood, 2001).
- Wernicke's encephalopathy describes an acute state of confusion, ataxia, and abnormal eye movements that are related to thiamine deficiency (Rigler, 2000).
- Alcohol can inflame the stomach lining and impede the body's ability to absorb vitamins.
- Korsakoff's syndrome is caused by the tendency for inadequate nutrition to accompany chronic alcoholism, thus resulting in a number of vitamin deficiencies and metabolic changes (Menninger, 2002).

- Older adults' mentation may improve as superimposed delirium clears with abstinence, but residual deficits in memory and judgment are common (Smith, 1995).

Sleep Deprivation. Reduced phase IV or deep sleep that accompanies normal aging results in very little deep sleep for the elderly alcoholic (Brower & Hall, 2001).

Skeletal Problems. Alcohol problems exacerbate neuromuscular issues.

- Older adults are predisposed to falls when the postural support mechanism is lost (Rigler, 2000).
- Osteoporosis, combined with the detrimental effects of alcohol on gait and balance, results in higher age-adjusted rates of hip fracture among older alcoholic patients (American Medical Association, 1996).
- Older adults with alcohol-related disease were found to have a 2.6-fold increased risk of hip fracture compared with older adults without alcohol-related disease, and a higher mortality one year later (Yuan, Dawson, Cooper, Einstadter, Cebul, & Rimm, 2001).

Organ System Problems. Alcohol has adverse effects on all organ systems (Smith, 1995).

- Gastrointestinal disease and bleeding are common reasons for emergency department visits by older alcoholic patients (Adams, Magruder-Habib, Trued, & Broome, 1992).
- Elevated liver enzymes are found in 18% of older alcoholics (Hurt, Finlayson, Morse, & Davis, 1988) and may indicate alcoholic hepatitis, fatty liver, or cirrhosis. Half of older adults with cirrhosis die within one year of diagnosis (Smith, 1995).
- Moderate drinking may exacerbate hypertension and heavy drinking increases the risk of stroke.
- Older adults who abuse alcohol are at risk for immunosuppression and, thus, are at increased risk of infection.
- Many older adults were exposed to tuberculosis during childhood, and physicians should remain vigilant for reactivated disease in older alcoholic patients.

Assessment

Ideally, assessment of substance use should include multiple sources of information (e.g., collateral sources such as family, medical records) prior to the development of a treatment plan. A detailed assessment is often not practical and clinicians may have to rely on a single brief interview. Given practical constraints, it is recommended that clinicians focus on obtaining a detailed description of the individual's current level of use and the context in which it occurs. The assessment should include a history and severity of use; the short- and long-term emotional (e.g., avoidance and escape from negative emotions), social, and lifestyle (e.g., reduced financial resources) consequences of substance use; current social support; barriers to treatment (e.g., personal barriers such as rationalizing and practical such as transportation); motivation and readiness to change; life stressors; comorbid mental or physical health problems (including chronology); previous treatment attempts; risk factors for relapse; and personal strengths (e.g., problem-solving skills, religious faith) (Marlatt & Witkiewitz, 2006).

The most commonly utilized screening instrument for alcohol drinking problems in older adults is the CAGE (Buchsbaum, Buchanan, Welsh, Centor, & Schnoll, 1992). The CAGE can effectively discriminate older patients with a history of drinking problems from those without such a history with four simple questions: C—Have you ever felt you should cut down on your drinking? A—Have people annoyed you by criticizing your drinking? G—Have you ever felt guilty about your drinking? E—Have you ever had a drink first thing in the morning (i.e., an eye-opener)?

Prescription and Over-the-Counter Drug Abuse

Older adults are at high risk for medication-related adverse events due to the large number of prescription medications and age-related physiologic changes in pharmacokinetics and pharmacodynamics (Patterson, Lacro, & Jeste, 1999). On average, older adults take three to five prescription medications per day (Williams, 2002). Medication misuse may include overuse because of a belief that more is better and underuse due to cost issues or as a method to avoid side effects. Abuse of prescribed or over-the-counter (OTC) drugs occurs when a patient continues to use the drug even when it is not required for the primary purpose for which it was recommended, or when the person takes it in greater than recommended amounts because of its psychotropic effects (Patterson, Lacro, & Jeste, 1999). Accurate estimates of the prevalence of prescription and OTC drug abuse in the elderly are not available, with estimates ranging from 5% to 33% (Jinks & Raschko, 1990; Ostrum et al., 1985).

Evidence-Based Interventions for Substance Abuse

While very little research has been conducted on the treatment of substance abuse with older adults, studies do indicate that older adults benefit from formal substance abuse treatment. Older adults stay in treatment longer and have outcomes at least as favorable as younger adults in mixed-age programs (Atkinson, Tolson & Turner, 1993; Satre, Mertens, Arean, & Weisner, 2003). Older patients may gain additional treatment benefits from elder-specific programs (Blow, Walton, Chermack, Mudd, & Brower, 2000). Unfortunately, many older adults who could benefit from services appear to encounter treatment initiation and access barriers. Treatment entry rates among medically ill middle-age and older adults are low (e.g., 10–15%; Stephan, Swindle & Moos, 1992), suggesting that many older adults are not receiving the treatment they need.

Pharmacological Treatments

Research findings provide little evidence supporting the effectiveness of pharmacological interventions for geriatric substance abuse (Schonfeld & Dupree, 1995; American Medical Association, 1996; Fingerhood, 2000).

Psychological Treatments

Psychological treatment for substance use disorders can be conducted individually or in groups; in outpatient or inpatient settings; as aftercare following inpatient treatment (e.g., relapse prevention programs); and as brief interventions (Miller, Rollnick, & Con, 2002; Moyer, Finney, Swearingen, & Vergun, 2002). Effective treatment components for older adults include treatment groups exclusively for older persons, supportive and nonconfrontational treatment approaches, and group or individual cognitive behavioral therapy (Gatz et al., 1998).

Behavior Therapy. Individual behavior therapy and behavioral marital therapy are effective treatments for patients with substance abuse disorders (Higgins et al., 1991; Holder, Longabaugh, Miller, & Rubonis, 1991; Miller & Hester, 1986; see Marlatt & Witkiewitz, 2006 for a review of the evidence based interventions). Superior outcomes result from community reinforcement counseling plus incentives compared with 12-step counseling alone (Higgins et al., 1991; Higgins et al., 1994). Contingency contracting has shown positive outcomes during the period when the contract is in effect, promoting treatment compliance and abstinence. In one study, the addition of contingency-based counseling, general medical care, and psychosocial services improved the efficacy of methadone maintenance treatment in newly admitted opioid patients (McLellan, Arndt, Metzger, Woody, & O'Brien, 1993). Urine toxicology testing to monitor for illicit drug use and provision of rewards for abstinence or aversive consequences for illicit drug use has also been effective (Brahen, Henderson, Capone, & Kordal, 1984; Vaillant, 1988; Stitzer, Iguchi, & Felch, 1992).

Cognitive Behavioral Therapy. Cognitive behavioral treatments aimed at improving self-control, emotional coping, and social skills have been found to be effective for reducing alcohol abuse (Holder, Longabaugh, Miller, & Rubonis, 1991; Chaney, 1989; Monti et al., 1990). Self-control strategies include goal setting, self-monitoring, functional analysis of drinking antecedents, and learning alternative coping skills.

Social skills training focuses on learning skills for forming and maintaining interpersonal relationships, assertiveness, and drink refusal. Cognitive therapy interventions that are focused on identifying and modifying maladaptive thoughts without a behavioral component have not been found to be as effective as cognitive behavioral treatments (Holder et al., 1991).

REFERENCE AND RESOURCE LIST

Adams, W. L., Barry, K. L., & Fleming, M. F. (1996). Screening for problem drinking in older primary care patients. *Journal of the American Medical Associations, 276,* 1964–1967.

Adams, W. L., Magruder-Habib, K., Trued, S., & Broome, H. L. (1992). Alcohol abuse in elderly emergency department patients. *Journal of the American Geriatrics Society, 40*(12), 1236–1240.

Alwahhabi, F. (2003). Anxiety symptoms and generalized anxiety disorder in the elderly: A review. *Harvard Review of Psychiatry, 11*(4), 180–193.

American Medical Association. (1996). Council on Scientific Affairs of the American Medical Association: Alcoholism in the elderly. *Journal of the American Medical Association, 275,* 797–801.

American Psychiatric Association. (1994). *Diagnostic and statistical manual of mental disorders* (4th ed.). Washington, DC: Author.

American Psychiatric Association. (2000). *Diagnostic and statistical manual of mental disorders* (4th ed., text revision). Washington, DC: Author.

Antony, M. M. (2001). Assessment of anxiety and the anxiety disorders: An overview. In M. M. Antony, S. M. Orsillo & L. Roemer (Eds.), *Practitioner's guide to empirically based measures of anxiety (pp. 9–18).* New York: Kluwer Academic/Plenum Publishers.

Areán, P. A. (2004). Psychosocial treatments for depression in the elderly. *Primary Psychiatry, 11*(5), 48–53.

Areán, P. A., & Alvidrez, J. (2001). The prevalence of psychiatric disorders and subsyndromal mental illness in low-income, medically ill elderly. *International Journal of Psychiatry in Medicine, 31*(1), 9–24.

Ashendorf, L., Constantinou, M., & McCaffrey, R. J. (2004). The effect of depression and anxiety on the TOMM in community-dwelling older adults. *Archives of Clinical Neuropsychology, 19*(1), 125–130.

Atkinson, R. M., Tolson, R. L., & Turner, J. A. (1993). Factors affecting outpatient treatment compliance of older male problem drinkers. *Journal of Studies on Alcohol, 54,* 102–106.

Averill, P. M., & Beck, J. G. (2000). Posttraumatic stress disorder in older adults: A conceptual review. *Journal of Anxiety Disorders, 14*(2), 133–156.

Bartels, S. J., Blow, F. C., Brockmann, L. M., & Van Citters, A. D. (2005). *Substance abuse and mental health among older Americans: The state of the knowledge and future directions.* Rockville, MD: Older American Substance Abuse and Mental Health Technical Assistance Center, Substance Abuse and Mental Health Services Administration.

Beck, A. T., & Steer, R. A. (1993). *Beck anxiety inventory: Manual* (2nd ed.). San Antonio, TX: Psychological Corporation.

Beck, A. T., Rush, A. J., Shaw, B. F., & Emery, G. (1979). *Cognitive therapy of depression.* New York: The Guilford Press.

Beck, A. T., Steer, R. A., & Brown, G. K. (1996). *Beck depression inventory II manual.* San Antonio, TX: The Psychological Corporation.

Beck, J. G., & Stanley, M. A. (2001). Assessment of anxiety disorders in older adults: Current concerns, future prospects. In M. M. Antony, S. M. Orsillo & L. Roemer (Eds.), *Practitioner's guide to empirically based measures of anxiety* (pp. 43–48). New York: Kluwer Academic/Plenum Publishers.

Beekman, A. T. F., Deeg, D. J. H., Van Limbeek, J., & Braam, A. W. (1997). Criterion validity of the Center for Epidemiologic Studies Depression scale (CES-D): Results from a community-based sample of older subjects in the Netherlands. *Psychological Medicine, 27*(1), 231–235.

Blake, D. D., Weather, F. W., Nagy, L. M., Kaloupek, D. G., Gusman, F. D., Charney, D. S., et al. (1995). The development of a clinician-administered PTSD scale. *Journal of Traumatic Stress, 8,* 75–90.

Blake, D. D., Weathers, F. W., Nagy, L. M., Kaloupek, D. G., Klauminzer, G., Charney, D. S., et al. (1990). A clinician rating scale for assessing current and lifetime PTSD: The CAPS-1. *The Behavior Therapist, 13,* 187–188.

Blow, F., Walton, M. , Chermack, S., Mudd, S., & Brower, K. (2000). Older adult treatment outcome following elder-specific inpatient alcoholism treatment. *Journal of Substance Abuse Treatment, 19*(1), 67–75.

Brahen, L. S., Henderson, R. K., Capone, T., & Kordal, N. (1984). Naltrexone treatment in a jail work-release program. *Journal of Clinical Psychiatry, 45,* 49–52.

Briere, J. (1995). *Trauma Symptom Inventory professional manual.* Odessa, FL: Psychological Assessment Resources.

Briere, J., Elliot, D. M., Harris, K., & Cotman, A. (1995). Trauma Symptom Inventory: Psychometrics and association with childhood and adult victimization in clinical samples. *Journal of Interpersonal Violence, 10*(4), 387–401.

Brower, K. J., & Hall, J. M. (2001). Effects of age and alcoholism on sleep: A controlled study. *Journal of Studies on Alcohol, 62*(3), 335–343.

Brown, T. A., DiNardo, P., & Barlow, D. H. (1994). *Anxiety disorders interview schedule adult version (ADIS—IV): Client interview schedule.* Albany, NY: Graywind Publications.

Brown, T. A., O'Leary, T. A., & Barlow, D. H. (2001). Generalized anxiety disorder. In D. H. Barlow (Ed.), *Clinical handbook of psychological disorders: A step-by-step treatment manual* (3rd ed.). New York: The Guilford Press.

Buchsbaum, D. G., Buchanan, R. G., Welsh, J., Centor, R., & Schnoll, S. (1992). Screening for drinking disorders in the elderly using the CAGE questionnaire. *Journal of the American Geriatrics Society, 40*(7), 662–667.

Burns, D. D. (1999a). *Feeling good: The new mood therapy* (2nd ed.). New York: Avon Books.

Burns, D. D. (1999b). *The feeling good handbook.* New York: Plume.

Busuttil, W. (2004). Presentation and management of post traumatic stress disorder and the elderly: A need for investigation. *International Journal of Geriatric Psychiatry, 19,* 429–439.

Calamari, J. E., Faber, S. D., Hitsman, B L., & Poppe, C. J. (1994). Treatment of obsessive-compulsive disorder in the elderly: A review and case example. *Journal of Behavior Therapy and Experimental Psychiatry, 25,* 95–104.

Chaney, E. F. (1989). Social skills training. In R. K. Hester & W. R. Miller (Eds.), *Handbook of alcoholism treatment approaches* (pp. 206–221). New York: Pergamon Press.

Cook, J. M., Areán, P. A., Schnurr, P. P., & Sheikh, J. I. (2001). Symptom differences between older depressed primary care patients with and without history of trauma. *International Journal of Psychiatry in Medicine, 31*(4), 410–414.

Coon, D. W., Thompson, L., Steffen, A., Sorocco, K., & Gallagher-Thompson, D. (2003). Anger and depression management: Psychoeducational skills training interventions for women caregivers of a relative with dementia. *Gerontologist, 43*(5), 678–689.

Craske, M. G., & Barlow, D. H. (2001). Panic disorder and agoraphobia. In D. H. Barlow (Ed.), *Clinical handbook of psychological disorders: A step-by-step treatment manual* (3rd ed., pp. 1–59). New York: The Guilford Press.

de Beurs, E., Beekman, A. T., van Balkom, A. J., Deeg, D. J., van Dyck, R., & van Tilburg, W. (1999). Consequences of anxiety in older persons: Its effect on disability, well-being and use of health services. *Psychological Medicine, 29,* 583–593.

Derogatis, L. R., Lipman, R. S., Rickels, K., Uhlenhuth, E. H., & Covi, L. (1974). The Hopkins symptom checklist (HSCL): A self-report symptom inventory. *Behavioral Science, 19,* 1–15.

Dew, M. A., Reynolds, C. F., Mulsant, B., Frank, E., Houck, P. R., Matzumdar, S., et al. (2001). Initial recovery patterns may predict which maintenance therapies for depression will keep older adults well. *Journal of Affective Disorders, 65,* 155–166.

Dobson, K. S., & Hamilton, K. E. (2003). Cognitive restructuring: Behavioral tests of negative conditions. In W. O'Donohue, J. E. Fisher & S. C. Hayes (Eds.), *Cognitive behavior therapy: Applying empirically supported techniques in your practice* (pp. 84–88). Hoboken, NJ: Wiley.

Draper, B. (1996). Attempted suicide in old age. *International Journal of Geriatric Psychiatry, 11,* 577–587.

Ellis, A. (2003). Cognitive restructuring of the disputing of irrational beliefs. In W. O'Donohue, J. E. Fisher & S. C. Hayes (Eds.), *Cognitive behavior therapy: Applying empirically supported techniques in your practice* (pp. 79–83). Hoboken, NJ: Wiley.

Erickson, C. L., & Muramatsu, N. (2004). Parkinson's disease, depression and medication adherence: Current knowledge and social work practice. *Journal of Gerontological Social Work, 42*(3–4), 3–18.

Fabian, L. J., & Haley, W. E. (1991). Behavioral treatment of claustrophobia in a geriatric patient: A case study. *Clinical Gerontologist, 10,* 15–22.

Feeney, S. L. (2004). The relationship between pain and negative affect in older adults: Anxiety as a predictor of pain. *Anxiety Disorders, 18,* 733–744.

Ferguson, K. L. (2003). Relaxation. In W. O'Donohue, J. E. Fisher & S. C. Hayes (Eds.), *Cognitive behavior therapy: Applying empirically supported techniques in your practice* (pp. 330–340). Hoboken, NJ: Wiley.

Fingerhood, M. (2000). Substance abuse in older people. *Journal of the American Geriatrics Society, 48,* 985–995.

First, M. B., Spitzer, R. L., Gibbon, M., & Williams, J. B. W. (1996). *Structured clinical interview for DSM-IV axis I disorders—Patient edition* (SCID-I/P, Version 2.0). New York: Biometrics Research Department, New York State Psychiatric Institute.

First, M. B., Spitzer, R. L., Gibbon, M., & Williams, J. B. W. (1997). *Structured clinical interview for DSM-IV axis I disorders—Clinical version* (SCID-CV). Washington, DC: American Psychiatric Press.

Foa, E. B., Cashman, L. A., Jaycox, L., & Perry, K. (1997). The validation of a self-report measure of posttraumatic stress disorder: The Posttraumatic Diagnostic Scale. *Psychological Assessment, 4,* 445–451.

Foa, E. B., Keane, T. M., & Friedman, M. J. (Eds.) (2000). *Effective treatments for PTSD: Practice guidelines from the International Society for Traumatic Stress Studies.* New York: Guilford Press.

Forsyth, J. P., & Fusé, T. (2003). Interoceptive exposure for panic disorder. In W. O'Donohue, J. E. Fisher & S. C. Hayes (Eds.), *Cognitive behavior therapy: Applying empirically supported techniques in your practice* (pp. 212–222). Hoboken, NJ: Wiley.

Free, M. L. (1999). *Cognitive therapy in groups: Guidelines and resources for practice.* Chichester. U.K.: Wiley.

Fuentes, K., & Cox, B. J. (1997). Prevalence of anxiety disorders in elderly adults: A critical analysis. *Journal of Behavior Therapy and Experimental Psychiatry, 28*(4), 269–279.

Gallagher-Thompson, D., Haley, W. E., Guy, D., Rubert, M., Arguelles, T., Tennstedt, S., et al. (2003). Tailoring psychosocial interventions for ethnically diverse dementia caregivers. *Clinical Psychology: Science and Practice, 10*, 423–438.

Gallagher-Thompson, D., Lovett, S., Rose, J., McKibbin, C., Coon, D., Futterman, A., et al. (2000). Impact of psychoeducational interventions on distressed family caregivers. *Journal of Clinical Geropsychology, 6*, 91–110.

Garber, J., & Flynn, C. (2001). Vulnerability to depression in childhood and adolescence. In R. E. Ingram & J. M. Price (Eds.), *Vulnerability to psychopathology: Risk across the lifespan* (pp. 175–225). New York: Guilford.

Garfinkel, R. (1979). Brief behavior therapy with an elderly patient: A case study. *Journal of Geriatric Psychiatry, 12*, 101–109.

Gatz, M., Fiske, A., Fox, L. S., Kaskie, B., Kasl-Godley, J. E., McCallum, T. J., et al., (1998). Empirically validated psychological treatments for older adults. *Journal of Mental Health and Aging, 4*, 9–46.

Goldberg, J. H., Breckenridge, J. N., & Sheikh, J. I. (2003). Age differences in symptoms of depression and anxiety: Examining behavioral medicine outpatients. *Journal of Behavioral Medicine, 26*(2), 119–132.

Gomberg, E. S. (1995). Older women and alcohol use and abuse. In M. Galanter (Ed.), *Recent developments in alcoholism: volume 12. Alcoholism and women* (pp. 61–79). New York: Plenum Press.

Graham, C., Arthur, A., & Howard, R. (2002). The social functioning of older adults with schizophrenia. *Aging & Mental Health, 6*(2), 149–152.

Gray, S. L., Lai, K. V., & Larson, E. B. (1999). Drug-induced cognition disorders in the elderly: Incidence, prevention, and management. *Drug Safety, 21*(2), 101–122.

Hamblin, D. L., Beutler, L., Scogin, F., & Corbishley, A. (1993). Patient responsiveness to therapist values and outcome in group cognitive therapy. *Psychotherapy Research, 3*(1), 36–46.

Hamilton, M. (1959). The assessment of anxiety states. *British Journal of Medical Psychology, 32*, 50–55.

Hamilton, M. (1960). A rating scale for depression. *Journal of Neurology, Neurosurgery and Psychiatry, 23*, 56–62.

Harwood, D. G., Barker, W. W., Ownby, R. L., Mullan, M., & Duara, R. (2004). No association between subjective memory complaints and apolipoprotein E genotype in cognitively intact elderly. *International Journal of Geriatric Psychiatry, 19*(12), 1131–1139.

Hazlett-Stevens, H., & Craske, M. G. (2003). Live (in vivo) exposure. In W. O'Donohue, J. E. Fisher & S. C. Hayes (Eds.), *Cognitive behavior therapy: Applying empirically supported techniques in your practice* (pp. 223–228). Hoboken, NJ: Wiley.

Head, L. S., & Gross, A. M. (2003). Systematic desensitization. In W. O'Donohue, J. E. Fisher & S. C. Hayes (Eds.), *Cognitive behavior therapy: Applying empirically supported techniques in your practice* (pp. 417–422). Hoboken, NJ: Wiley.

Herbert, J. D., & Forman, E. M. (in press). Posttraumatic stress disorder. In J. E. Fisher & W. O'Donohue (Eds.), *Practice guidelines for evidence-based psychotherapy*. New York: Springer Publishing.

Higgins, S. T., Budney, A. J., Bickel, W. K., Foerg, F. E., Donham, R., & Badger, G. J. (1994). Incentives improve outcome in outpatient behavioral treatment of cocaine dependence. *Archives of General Psychiatry, 51,* 568–576.

Higgins, S. T., Delaney, D. D., Budney, A. J., Bickel, W. K., Hughes, J. R., Foerg, F., et al. (1991). A behavioral approach to achieving initial cocaine abstinence. *American Journal of Psychiatry, 148,* 1218–1224.

Holder, H. D., Longabaugh, R., Miller, W. R., & Rubonis, A. V. (1991). The cost effectiveness of treatment for alcoholism: A first approximation. *Journal of Studies on Alcoholism, 52,* 517–540.

Howard, R., & Bandyopadhyay, D. (1993). Selective serotonin reuptake inhibitors for the elderly. *International Journal of Geriatric Psychiatry, 8,* 627–629.

Hunt, G. M., & Azrin, N. H. (1973). A community reinforcement approach to alcoholism. *Behavior Research and Therapy, 11,* 91–104.

Hurt, R. D., Finlayson, R. E., Morse, R. M., & Davis, L. J., Jr. (1988). Alcoholism in elderly persons: Medical aspects and prognosis of 216 inpatients. *Mayo Clinic Proceedings, 63,* 753–60.

Jinks, M. J., & Raschko, R. R. (1990). A profile of alcohol and prescription drug abuse in a high-risk community-based elderly population. *DICP, 24*(10), 971–975.

Joseph, C. L., Ganzini, L., & Atkinson, R. M. (1995). Screening for alcohol use disorders in the nursing home. *Journal of the American Geriatrics Society, 43*(4), 368–373.

Junginger, J., & Ditto, B. (1984). Multitreatment of obsessive-compulsive checking in a geriatric patient. *Behavior Modification, 8,* 379–390.

Kane, R. L. (2000). Choosing and using an assessment tool. In R. L. Kane & R. A. Kane (Eds.), *Assessing older persons: Measures, meaning, and practical implications* (pp. 1–13). New York: Oxford University Press, Inc.

Kogan, J. N., Edelstein, B. A., & McKee, D. R. (2000). Assessment of anxiety in older adults: Current status. *Journal of Anxiety Disorders, 14*(2), 109–132.

Kollins, S. H., Ehrhardt, K., & Poling, A. (2000). Clinical drug assessment. In A. Poling & T. Byrne (Eds.), *Introduction to behavioral pharmacology* (pp. 191–218). Reno, NV: Context Press.

Kril, J. J., Halliday, G. M., Svoboda, M. D., & Cartwright, H. (1997). The cerebral cortex is damaged in chronic alcoholics. *Neuroscience, 79*(4), 983–998.

Kudoh, A., Takase, H., Takahira, Y., & Takazawa, T. (2004). Postoperative confusion increases in elderly long-term benzodiazepine users. *Anesthesia & Analgesia, 99*(6), 1674–1678.

Lewinsohn, P. M., Munoz, R. F., Youngren, M. A., & Zeiss, A. M. (1992). *Control your depression*. New York: Fireside/Simon & Schuster.

Liang, J., Tran, T. V., Krause, N., & Markides, K. S. (1989). Generational differences in the structure of the CES-D in Mexican-Americans. *Journal of Gerontology, 44,* S110–S120.

Liberto, J. G., & Oslin, D. W. (1995). Early versus late onset of alcoholism in the elderly. *International Journal of Addictions, 30,* 1799–1818.

Lombardo, T. W., & Gray, M. J. (2005). Beyond exposure for posttraumatic stress disorder (PTSD) symptoms. *Behavior Modification, 29*(1), 3–9.

Longo, L. P., & Johnson, B. (2000). Addiction: Part I. Benzodiazepines—side effects, abuse risk and alternatives. *American Family Physician, 61,* 2121–2128.

Luoma, J. B., & Hayes, S. C. (2003). Cognitive defusion. In W. O'Donohue, J. E. Fisher & S. C. Hayes (Eds.), *Cognitive behavior therapy: Applying empirically supported techniques in your practice* (pp. 71–78). Hoboken, NJ: Wiley.

Marks, I. M., & Matthews, A. M. (1979). Brief standard self-rating for phobic patients. *Behaviour Research and Therapy, 17,* 263–267.

Marlatt, G. A., & Witkiewitz, K. (in press). Substance use disorders. In J. E. Fisher, & W. O'Donohue (Eds.), *Practice guidelines for evidence-based psychotherapy.* New York: Springer Publishing.

Martell, C. R., Addis, M., & Jacobson, N. (2001). *Depression in context: Strategies for guided action.* New York: Norton & Company.

Masters, J. C., Burish, T. G., Hollon, S., D., & Rimm, D. C. (1987). *Behavior therapy: Techniques and empirical findings (3rd ed.).* Fort Worth: Harcourt Brace Jovanovich.

McLellan, A. T., Arndt, I. O., Metzger, D. S., Woody, G. E., & O'Brien, C. P. (1993). The effects of psychological services in substance abuse treatment. *Journal of the American Medical Association, 269,* 1953–1959.

Menninger, J. A. (2002). Assessment and treatment of alcoholism and substance-related disorders in the elderly [Electronic version]. *Bulletin of the Menninger Clinic, 66*(2).

Meyer, R. E., & Mirin, S. M. (1991). A psychology of craving: implications of behavioral research. In J. H. Lowinson & P. Ruiz (Eds.), *Substance abuse: Clinical problems and perspectives* (pp. 57–62). Baltimore: Williams & Wilkins.

Meyer, T. J., Miller, M. L., Metzger, R. L., & Borkovec, T. D. (1990). Development and validation of the Penn State Worry Questionnaire. *Behaviour Research and Therapy, 28,* 487–495.

Miller, W. R., & Hester, R. K. (1986). Inpatient treatment for alcoholism: Who benefits? *American Psychologist, 41,* 794–805.

Miller, W. R., Rollnick, S., & Con, K. (2002). *Motivational interviewing: Preparing people for change* (2nd ed.). New York: Guilford Press.

Mirand, A. L., & Welte, J. W. (1996). Alcohol consumption among the elderly in a general population, Erie County, New York. *American Journal of Public Health, 86,* 978–984.

Mittman, N., Herrmann, N., Einarson, T. R., Busto, U. E., Lanctot, L., Liu, B. A., et al. (1997). The efficacy, safety, and tolerability of antidepressants in late life depression: A meta-analysis. *Journal of Affective Disorders, 46,* 191–217.

Mohlman, J. (2004). Psychosocial treatment of late-life generalized anxiety disorder: Current status and future directions. *Clinical Psychology Review, 24,* 149–169.

Mojtabai, R., & Olfson, M. (2004). Cognitive deficits and course of major depression in a cohort of middle-aged and older community-dwelling adults. *Journal of the American Geriatric Society, 52*(7), 1060–1069.

Monti, P. M., Abrams, D. B., Binkoff, J. A., Zwick, W. R., Liepman, M. R., Nirenberg, T. D., et al. (1990). Communication skills training, communication skills training with family and cognitive behavioral mood management training for alcoholics. *Journal of Studies on Alcoholism, 51,* 263–270.

Moyer A., Finney J. W., Swearingen C. E., & Vergun P. (2002). Brief interventions for alcohol problems: A meta-analytic review of controlled investigations in treatment-seeking and non-treatment-seeking populations. *Addiction, 97,* 279–292.

Newman, C. F. (2003). Cognitive restructuring: Identifying and modifying maladaptive schemas. In W. O'Donohue, J. E. Fisher & S. C. Hayes (Eds.), *Cognitive behavior therapy: Applying empirically supported techniques in your practice* (pp. 59–64). Hoboken, NJ: Wiley.

Nordhus, I. H., & Pallesen, S. (2003). Psychological treatment of late-life anxiety: An empirical review. *Journal of Consulting and Clinical Psychology, 71*(4), 643–651.

Orsillo, S. M., Batten, S. V., & Hammond, C. (2001). Acute stress disorder and posttraumatic stress disorder: A brief overview and guide to assessment. In M. M. Antony, S. M. Orsillo, & L. Roemer (Eds.) *Practitioner's guide to empirically based measures of anxiety* (pp. 245–252). New York: Kluwer Academic/Plenum Publishers.

Öst, L. G. (1989). One-session treatment for specific phobias. *Behaviour Research and Therapy, 27*(1), 1–7.

Ostrom, J. R., Hammarlund, E. R., Christensen, D. B., Plein, J. B., Kethley, A. J., et al. (1985). Medication usage in an elderly population. *Medical Care, 23*(2), 157–164.

Padala, P. R., Roccaforte, W. H., & Burke, W. J. (2004). Antidepressants in the treatment of depression in older adults. *Primary Psychiatry, 11*(8), 35–39.

Paterniti, S., Dufouil, C., & Alperovitch, A. (2002). Long-term benzodiazepine use and cognitive decline in the elderly: The Epidemiology of Vascular Aging Study. *Journal of Clinical Psychopharmacology, 22*(3), 285–293.

Patterson, T. L., Lacro, J. P., & Jeste, D. V. (1999). Abuse and misuse of medications in the elderly [Electronic version]. *Psychiatric Times, 26*(4).

Preville, M., Cote, G., Boyer, R., & Hebert, R. (2004). Detection of depression and anxiety disorders by home care nurses. *Aging & Mental Health, 8*(5), 400–409.

Radloff, L. S. (1977). The CES-D scale: A self-report depression scale for research in the general population. *Applied Psychological Measurement, 1,* 385–401.

Rapp, S. R., Smith, S. S., & Britt, M. (1990). Identifying comorbid depression in elderly medical patients: Use of the Extracted Hamilton Depression Rating Scale. *Psychological Assessment, 2*(3), 243–247.

Rathus, J. H., & Sanderson, W. C. (1996). Cognitive-behavioral treatment of panic disorder in elderly adults: Two case studies. *Journal of Cognitive Psychotherapy: An International Quarterly, 10,* 271–280.

Rigler, S. K. (2000). Alcoholism in the elderly. *American Family Physician, 61,* 1710–1716.

Robins, L. N., Helzer, J. E., Croughan, J. L., & Ratcliff, K. S. (1981). National Institute of Mental Health Diagnostic Interview Schedule: Its history, characteristics, and validity. *Archives of General Psychiatry, 38,* 381–389.

Rothbaum, B. O., Hodges, L. F., Ready, D., Graap, K., & Alarcon, R. D. (2001). Virtual reality exposure therapy for Vietnam veterans with posttraumatic stress disorder. *Journal of Clinical Psychiatry, 62*(8), 617–622.

Rothbaum, B. O., Meadows, E., Resick, P., & Foy, D. W. (2000). Cognitive-behavioral therapy. In E. B. Foa, T. M. Keane, & M. J. Friedman (Eds.), *Effective treatments for PTSD: Practice guidelines from the International Society for Traumatic Stress Studies* (pp. 84–105). New York: Guilford Press.

Rothschild, A. J. (1996). The diagnosis and treatment of late-life depression. *Journal of Clinical Psychiatry, 57*(Suppl. 5), 5–11.

Rowan, V. C., Holburn, S. W., Walker, J. R., & Siddiqui, A. R. (1984). A rapid multicomponent treatment for obsessive-compulsive disorder. *Journal of Behavior Therapy and Experimental Psychiatry, 15,* 347–352.

Ruscio, A. M., & Borkovec, T. D. (2004). Experience and appraisal of worry among high worriers with and without generalized anxiety disorder. *Behaviour Research and Therapy, 42,* 1469–1482.

Salzman, C. (2005). Treatment of anxiety and anxiety-related disorders. In C. Salzman (Ed.), *Clinical geriatric psychopharmacology* (4th ed. pp. 261–281). Philadelphia, PA: Lippincott Williams & Wilkins.

Salzman, C., & Sheikh, J. I. (2005). Diagnosis of anxiety and anxiety-related disorders. In C. Salzman (Ed.), *Clinical geriatric psychopharmacology* (4th ed. pp. 333–342). Philadelphia, PA: Lippincott Williams & Wilkins.

SAMSHA, Substance Abuse and Mental Health Services Administration. (2002). *National survey on drug use and health.* Rockville, MD: Author. Retrieved from at http://www.oas.samsha.gov.

SAMSHA, Substance Abuse and Mental Health Services Administration. (2005). *Substance use among older adults: 2002 and 2003 update.* Department of Health and Human Services, Office of Applied Statistics. Retrieved from http://www.oas.samsha.gov.

Sanavio, E. (1988). Obsessions and compulsions: The Padua Inventory. *Behaviour Research and Therapy, 26,* 169–197.

Satre, D. D., Mertens, J. M., Areán P. A., & Weisner, C. (2003). Contrasting outcomes of older versus middle-aged and younger adult chemical dependency patients in a managed care program. *Journal of Studies on Alcohol, 64,* 520–530.

Sawyer-Radloff, L., & Teri, L. (1986). Use of the Center for Epidemiological Studies-Depression Scale with older adults. *Clinical Gerontologist, 5,* 119–135.

Schonfeld, L., & Dupree, L. W. (1995). Treatment approaches for older problem drinkers. *International Journal of the Addictions, 30,* 1819–1842.

Schutte, K. K., Brennan, P. L., & Moos, R. H. (1994). Remission of late-life drinking problems: A 4-year follow-up. *Alcoholism: Clinical and Experimental Research, 18,* 835–844.

Scogin, F. (1987). The concurrent validity of the Geriatric Depression Scale with depressed older adults. *Clinical Gerontologist, 7*(1), 23–31.

Scogin, F. R., Rickard, H., Keith, S., Wilson, J., & McElreath, L. (1992). Progressive and imaginal relaxation training for elderly persons with subjective anxiety. *Psychology and Aging, 7*, 419–424.

Sheikh, J. I. (2004). Anxiolytics, sedatives, and older patients. *Primary Psychiatry, 11*(8), 51–54.

Sheikh, J. I., & Cassidy, E. L. (2000). Treatment of anxiety disorders in the elderly: Issues and strategies. *Journal of Anxiety Disorders, 14*(2), 173–190.

Sheikh, J. I., & Yesavage, J. A. (1986). Geriatric Depression Scale: Recent evidence and development of a shorter version. *Clinical Gerontologist, 5*, 165–172.

Sirey, J., Bruce, M. L., & Alexopolous, G. S. (2005). Treatment initiation program: An intervention to improve depression outcomes among older adults. *American Journal of Psychiatry, 162*(1), 184–186.

Smith, J. W. (1995). Medical manifestations of alcoholism in the elderly. *International Journal of the Addictions, 30*(13–14), 1749–1798.

Sood, J. R., Cisek, E., Zimmerman, J., Zaleski, E. H., & Filmore, H. H. (2003). Treatment of depressive symptoms during short-term rehabilitation: An attempted replication of the DOUR project. *Rehabilitation Psychology, 48*(1), 44–49.

Spiegel, D. A., & Bruce, T. J. (1997). Benzodiazepines and exposure-based cognitive behavior therapies for panic disorder: Conclusions from combined treatment trials. *American Journal of Psychiatry, 154*, 773–781.

Spielberger, C. D., Gorsuch, R., Lushene, R., Vagg, P. R., & Jacobs, G. A. (1983). *STAI manual for the State-Trait Anxiety Inventory.* Palo Alto, CA: Consulting Psychologists Press.

Spitzer, R. L., Williams, J. B., Kroenke, K., Linzer, M., deGruy, F. V., III, Hahn, S. R., et al. (1995). Utility of a new procedure for diagnosing mental disorders in primary care. The PRIME-MD 1000 study. *American College of Physicians, 122*(3), 73.

Stanley, M. A., & Novy, D. M. (2000). Cognitive-behavior therapy for generalized anxiety in late life: An evaluative overview. *Journal of Anxiety Disorders, 14*(2), 191–207.

Stanley, M. A., Novy, D. M., Bourland, S. L., Beck, J. G., & Averill, P. M. (2001). Assessing older adults with generalized anxiety: A replication and extension. *Behaviour Research and Therapy, 39*, 221–235.

Stefanis, C. N., & Stefanis, N. C. (1999). Diagnosis of depressive disorders: A review. In M. Maj & N. Sartorius (Eds.), *Depressive Disorders* (pp. 1–51). New York: Wiley.

Stephan, M., Swindle, R. W., & Moos, R. H. (1992). *Alcohol screening in the Department of Veterans Affairs Medical Centers.* Washington, DC: Department of Veterans Affairs.

Stewart, S. A. (2005). The effects of benzodiazepines on cognition. *Clinical Psychiatry, 66*(S2), 9–13.

Stitzer, M. L., Iguchi, M. Y., & Felch, L. J. (1992). Contingent take-home incentive: Effects on drug use of methadone maintenance patients. *Journal of Consulting and Clinical Psychology, 60*, 927–934.

Swales, P. J., Solfvin, J. F., & Sheikh, J. I. (1996). Cognitive-behavioral therapy in older panic disorder patients. *American Journal of Geriatric Psychiatry, 4,* 46–60.

Tamblyn, R., Abrahamowicz, M., du Berger, R., McLeod, P., & Bartlett, G. (2005). A 5-year prospective assessment of the risk associated with individual benzodiazepines and doses in new elderly users. *Journal of the American Geriatrics Society, 53*(2), 233–241.

Thomas, V. S., & Rockwood, K. J. (2001). Alcohol abuse, cognitive impairment, and mortality among older people. *Journal of the American Geriatrics Society, 49*(4), 415–420.

Thyer, B. A. (1981). Prolonged in vivo exposure therapy with a 70-year old woman. *Journal of Behavior Therapy and Experimental Psychiatry, 12,* 69–71.

Turk, C. L., Heimberg, R. G., & Hope, D. A. (2001). Social anxiety disorder. In D. H. Barlow (Ed.), *Clinical handbook of psychological disorders: A step-by-step treatment manual* (3rd ed. pp. 114–153). New York: Guilford Press.

Turner, S. M., Hersen, M., Bellack, A. S., & Wells, K. C. (1979). Behavioral treatment of obsessive-compulsive neurosis. *Behaviour Research and Therapy, 17,* 95–106.

United States Department of Health and Human Services. (1999). *The Surgeon General's call to action to prevent suicide. At a glance: Suicide among the elderly.* Retrieved June 1, 2005, at http://www.surgeongeneral.gov/library/calltoaction/fact2.htm.

Unutzer, J., Katon, W., Callahan, C. M., William Jr., J. W., Hunkeler, E., Harpole, L., et al. (2003). Depression treatment in a sample of 1,801 depressed older adults in primary care. *Journal of the American Geriatrics Society, 51,* 505–514.

Vaillant, G. E. (1988). What can long-term follow-up teach us about relapse and prevention of relapse in addiction? *British Journal of Addiction, 83*(10), 1147–1157.

Verdoux, H., Lagnaoui, R., & Begaud, B. (2005). Is benzodiazepine use a risk factor for cognitive decline and dementia? A literature review of epidemiological studies. *Psychological Medicine, 35*(3), 307–315.

Wagner, A. W., Logsdon, R. G., Pearson, J. L., & Teri, L. (1997). Caregiver expressed emotion and depression in Alzheimer's disease. *Aging & Mental Health, 1*(2), 132–139.

Wanderer, Z. (1972). Existential depression treated by desensitization of phobias: Strategy and transcript. *Journal of Behavior Therapy and Experimental Psychiatry, 3,* 111–116.

Watson, L. C., Lewis, C. L., Kistler, C. E., Amick, H. R., & Boustani, M. (2004). Can we trust depression screening instruments in healthy "old-old" adults? *International Journal of Geriatric Psychiatry, 19*(3), 278–285.

Weathers, F. W., Ruscio, A. M., & Keane, T. M. (1999). Psychometric properties of nine scoring rules for the Clinician Administered Posttraumatic Stress Disorder Scale. *Psychological Assessment, 11,* 124–133.

Weintraub, D., & Ruskin, P. E. (1999). Posttraumatic stress disorder in the elderly: A review. *Harvard Review of Psychiatry, 7*(3), 144–152.

Wetherell, J. L. (1998). Treatment of anxiety in older adults. *Psychotherapy: Theory, Research, Practice, Training, 35*(4), 444–458.

Wetherell, J. L., & Gatz, M. (2005). The Beck Anxiety Inventory in older adults with generalized anxiety disorder. *Journal of Psychopathology and Behavioral Assessment, 27*(1), 17–24.

Williams, C. M. (2002). Using medications appropriately in older adults. *American Family Physician, 66*(10), 1917–1924.

Williams, M. J., Little, M. M., Scates, S., & Blockman, N. (1987). Memory complaints and abilities among depressed older adults. *Journal of Consulting and Clinical Psychology, 55*(4), 595–598.

Wisocki, P. A., Handen, B., & Morse, C. (1986). The Worry Scale as a measure of anxiety among homebound and community active elderly. *The Behavior Therapist, 5,* 91–95.

Wolpe, J., & Lazarus, A. A. (1966). *Behavior therapy techniques.* New York: Pergamon Press.

Yuan, Z., Dawson, N., Cooper, G. S., Einstadter, D., Cebul, R., & Rimm, A. A.(2001). Effects of alcohol-related disease on hip fracture and mortality: A retrospective cohort study of hospitalized Medicare beneficiaries. *American Journal of Public Health, 91*(7), 1089–1093.

Zauszniewski, J. A., Morris, D. L., Preechawong, S., & Chang, H. J. (2004). Reports on depressive symptoms in older adults with chronic conditions. *Research and Theory for Nursing Practice, 18*(2–3), 185–196.

Zung, W. (1971). A rating instrument for anxiety disorders. *Psychosomatics, 12,* 371–379.

CHAPTER 6

Evidence-Based Practices for Dementia and Schizophrenia

Jane E. Fisher, Kyle E. Ferguson, and Claudia Droßel

In this chapter we describe evidence-based assessment and treatment options for the care of elderly persons with dementia or schizophrenia. Both disorders result in significant impairment and the reliance of the person on caregivers. Treatment planning for persons with these problems should, therefore, be considered within the context of their social and physical environments. The need for case management support and family education emerges in early adulthood for persons with schizophrenia and continues throughout their lives. For persons with dementia, the (currently) inevitable loss of behaviors learned over a lifetime requires continuing assessment of the interaction of the person within the social and physical context.

DEMENTIA

Basic Facts About Dementia

Dementia is a descriptive term for a collection of symptoms that are caused by changes in brain function. Dementia can be caused by many conditions, some of which are reversible while others are not. Irreversible degenerative conditions such as Alzheimer's disease, vascular dementia, Lewy body disease, and frontal-temporal forms of dementia lead to progressive loss of cognitive functions. Other types of dementia can be halted or reversed with appropriate treatment. Reversible conditions that can cause symptoms of dementia include medication reactions, infection, metabolic disorders and endocrine abnormalities, dehydration, nutritional deficiencies, and subdural hematomas (National Institute of Neurological Diseases and Stroke, 2005).

Degenerative forms of dementia produce progressive declines in all intellectual abilities including memory, language, judgment, and abstract thinking. In advanced dementia, the development of challenging behaviors is common including physical and verbal aggression, disruptive vocalizations (e.g., screaming, repeating same question or sound hundreds of times a day), wandering, and public displays of sexual behavior. As persons become moderately to severely impaired, they require 24-hour supervision to ensure their safety. Persons with degenerative dementia eventually become completely dependent on others for their care. In the end stage of a degenerative dementia the person becomes bedridden, losing motor control including the ability to walk and swallow.

Estimates of the number of Americans with dementia range from 4 million to 6.8 million (National Institute on Aging, 2005). Estimates of the prevalence among persons over the age of 65 affected with dementia range from 10% to 20% (National Institute of Neurological Diseases and Stoke, 2005) to as high as 47% in persons over 85 (Evans et al., 1989). Age is the most important risk factor for dementia. The number of people with the disease doubles every 5 years beyond age 65. Dementia developing before the age of 65 ("early onset" dementia) is rare, accounting for 1–2% of cases (National Institute on Aging, 2005). The number of women diagnosed with dementia is greater than the number of men by a ratio of more than 2:1 due to the larger number of women who live to older ages when the risk of dementia is higher (Centers for Disease Control and Prevention, 1999).

The course and rate of decline varies significantly across patients. Stage models, which imply that the course of dementia occurs in an orderly fashion, have not been supported by empirical research. Persons with Alzheimer's disease live, on average, from 8 to 10 years after they are diagnosed, though the disease can last for as many as 20 years (National Institute on Aging, 2005).

Comorbidity

Persons with dementia are at high risk for chronic illnesses due to their age. Depression and anxiety are also highly prevalent in persons with dementia. It is estimated that up to 50% of persons with dementia experience depression (Forsell & Wingblad, 1998). Diagnosis of comorbid physical and psychological conditions can be difficult as verbal abilities decline and reporting of symptoms becomes impossible for the patient. Conditions associated with pain can be particularly problematic as the patient may not be able to report the source of pain.

Assessments

What Assessments Are Not Helpful?

Self-report measures normed on noncognitively impaired elderly populations may not be valid for use with a person with moderate or severe cognitive impairment. Traditional psychological tests such as the Minnesota Multiphasic Personality Inventory-2 (MMPI-2) (Butcher et al., 1989) and projective tests are not useful in assessing dementia.

What Is Involved in Effective Psychological Assessments?

1. *Rule out physical conditions* that might be causing or contributing to the problem. Conditions associated with chronic illnesses or acute pain (e.g., urinary tract infection, arthritis, indigestion, constipation), drug interactions or the side effects of commonly prescribed medications (e.g., nausea, sedation, dizziness, insomnia, agitation, fatigue, dry mouth, constipation, lightheadedness, headache, blurred vision, and confusion) should be ruled out prior to implementing a behavioral intervention for a person with dementia.

2. *Develop a precise behavioral description* (e.g., "moves from door to door turning door knobs for two hours in the afternoon" is more precise than "becomes agitated in the afternoon"). Direct observation methods are the most effective assessment strategies for describing the topography (including rate, frequency, duration, or severity) and identifying the context in which a specific problem behavior is occurring (see Bloom, Fischer, & Orme, 1995, for specific strategies).

Questionnaires such as the *Cohen-Mansfield Agitation Inventory* (Cohen-Mansfield & Billig, 1986) may be helpful for describing the topography and frequency of a problem behavior.

3. *Identify contingent relationships.* Descriptive ("Antecedent-Behavior-Consequence") analysis and an experimental (or functional) analysis are useful for identifying the function of problem behavior (i.e., the contingent relationship between problem behavior and environmental stimuli) (see Lerman & Iwata, 1993). Instruments useful for descriptive analyses of the function of a specific behavior problem include the Motivation Assessment Scale (MAS) (Durand & Crimmins, 1988); and the Functional Analysis Screening Tool (FAST) (Iwata, 1995).

4. *Design and implement behavioral intervention.* Behavioral interventions have been used to effectively increase adaptive behaviors (e.g., self-care

skills, verbal behavior) and decrease problem behaviors in elderly persons with dementia. A critical advantage of these interventions is that they preserve and promote the behavioral repertoire of persons with dementia whose repertoires were already greatly diminished due to the disease process. Numerous examples of the application of behavioral interventions for persons with dementia can be found in Burgio and Stevens (1999) and Fisher (in press).

Medical Assessments

The 1987 NIH Consensus Statement on the Diagnosis of Dementia emphasizes differentiation between progressive degenerative dementias (e.g., Alzheimer's type) and reversible dementia symptoms due to delirium, infection, metabolic or nutritional disorders, vascular system or cardiac disease, lesions, or normal pressure hydrocephalus. Early, accurate diagnosis of dementia is emphasized to allow early treatment of symptoms and the opportunity for the person with dementia to plan for the future while he or she can still participate in making decisions.

Confirmation of the accuracy of the diagnosis dementia requires an autopsy. Techniques recommended by the National Institute on Neurological Disorders and Stroke to help identify dementia with reasonable accuracy while the patient is still alive include

- *Patient history*, including how and when symptoms developed and the patient's overall medical condition.
- *Physical examination* to rule out treatable causes of dementia and to identify signs of stroke or other disorders that can contribute to dementia. Due to the high rate of prescription medications for diagnostic purposes, the NIH Consensus Statement recommends the withdrawal of all medications that are not absolutely necessary to see if the symptoms go away (NIH Consensus Statement Online, 1987; Stewart & Fairweather, 2002; see Gray, Kai, & Larson, 1999, for a review of drug-induced cognitive disorders in the elderly).
- *Neurological examination*, including assessment of balance, sensory functioning, reflexes, and other functions to identify signs of conditions (e.g., movement disorders or stroke) that may affect the patient's diagnosis or are treatable with medication.
- *Cognitive and neuropsychological tests* to assess memory, language skills, executive functions (such as problem solving), math skills, and other abilities related to mental functioning.

- *Brain scans* to identify evidence of brain atrophy, strokes, and transient ischemic attacks (TIAs), changes to the blood vessels, and other problems such as hydrocephalus and subdural hematomas that can cause dementia.
- *Laboratory tests* to rule out other conditions that can contribute to symptoms. A partial list of these tests includes a complete blood count, blood glucose test, urinalysis, drug and alcohol tests (toxicology screen), cerebrospinal fluid analysis (to rule out specific infections that can affect the brain), and analysis of thyroid and thyroid-stimulating hormone levels.

Evidence-Based Interventions for Dementia

Effective treatment planning for persons with dementia should consider patient characteristics (e.g., level of cognitive functioning, presence of challenging behavior), the support provided by the social and physical environments, and the dynamic interaction of the patient and environment as the disease progresses. The dependent relationship of the patient on others necessitates that treatment planning also target emotional and instrumental support for caregivers. Research has consistently demonstrated that caregivers of persons with dementia are at very high risk of negative effects on their own psychological and physical health (Pinquart & Sorenson, 2003; Schulz, O'Brien, Bookwala, & Fleissner, 1995). Support to enhance the functioning of the caregiver will directly benefit the person with dementia.

Psychotropic Drugs for Dementia

The main goal in the development of psychotropic drugs for dementia is to halt or at least slow the rate of deterioration. Psychotropic medication is also prescribed to reduce the frequency of challenging behaviors such as aggression, wandering, and disruptive vocalizations. In April of 2005 the Federal Drug Administration (FDA) issued a public health advisory to alert healthcare providers, patients, and patient caregivers to new safety information concerning an unapproved (i.e., "off-label") use of atypical antipsychotic drugs. Clinical studies of these drugs for the treatment of behavioral disorders in elderly patients with dementia have shown a higher death rate associated with their use compared to patients receiving a placebo. The advisory applies to atypical antipsychotic drugs including Abilify (aripiprazole), Zyprexa (olanzapine), Seroquel (quetiapine), Risperdal (risperidone), Clozaril (clozapine), and Geodon (ziprasidone).

The advisory is in response to an analysis of 17 placebo-controlled studies of four drugs in this class in which the rate of death for those elderly patients with dementia was found to about 1.6 to 1.7 times that of placebo. The FDA is also considering adding a warning to the labeling of older antipsychotic medications because limited data also suggest a similar increase in mortality for these drugs. Additional information concerning the advisory is available on FDA's Web site at http://www.fda.gov/cder/drug/infopage/antipsychotics/default.htm and at http://www.fda.gov/cder/drug/advisory/antipsychotics.htm.

Currently, there is no treatment that can reverse progressive degenerative dementia. The FDA has approved the use of five prescription drugs, which fall into the functional categories of acetylcholinesterase inhibitors for mild to moderate or N-methyl-D-asparate (NMDA) receptor antagonists for moderate to severe dementia of the Alzheimer's type (Cummings, 2004).

Acetylcholinesterase Inhibitors. By preventing the breakdown of acetylcholine acetylcholinesterase inhibitors enhance cholinergic neurotransmission. Recent evidence suggests that cholinergic drugs also affect dopaminergic systems (Zhang, Zhou, & Dani, 2004). The drugs in the following list differ in the selectivity with which they can inhibit cholinesterases, and increased selectivity correlates with fewer peripheral adverse effects (Sonkusare, Kaul, & Ramarao, 2005). Ranked in terms of general tolerability, donepezil leads, followed by galantamine and rivastigmine (Jones, 2003).

- Tacrine (Cognex˙, approved in 1993 and now rarely used; increased risk of hepatoxicity requires monitoring of liver transaminase.)
- Donepezil (Aricept˙, approved in 1996.)
- Rivastigmine (Exelon˙, approved in 2000.)
- Galantamine (Reminyl˙, approved in 2001.)

Acetylcholinesterase inhibitors have labeled indications for mild to moderate dementia of the Alzheimer's type and off-label use for other dementia subtypes (e.g., vascular dementia, dementia with Lewy body disease) as well as for attention-deficit hyperactivity disorder (ADHD), autism, and schizophrenia (Medline search, November, 2004).

Regarding effectiveness of acetylcholinesterase inhibitors, donepezil, galantamine, and rivastigmine are recommended as first-line pharmacological treatments of dementia by several professional groups (American Association for Geriatric Psychiatry, the Alzheimer's Association, the American Geriatrics Society, and the American Academy of Neurology). Recently, the effectiveness of acetylcholinesterase inhibitors, particularly of donepezil, has been questioned due to reported differences in benefits when administered in community settings with less well-defined, typical patients with high rates of comorbidity (Schneider, 2004) when compared with results from industry-sponsored randomized clinical trials (AD 2000 Collaborative Group, 2004; Jones, 2003; Kaduzkiewicz, Beck-Bornholdt, van den Bussche, & Zimmermann, 2004).

General information for donepezil, rivastigmine, and galantamine is available at www.aricept.com (donepezil); www.exelon.com (rivastigmine); www.reminyl.com (galantamine); and http://www.fda.gov/medwatch/SAFETY/2004/safety04.htm#Reminyl.

N-Methyl-D-Asparate (NMDA) Receptor Antagonists. The NMDA receptor antagonist, memantine, has been available in Europe as Akatinol® for the treatment of central nervous system disorders, multiple sclerosis, and mild to moderate dementia since 1982.* Memantine works on receptors sensitive to the effects of NMDA, a glutamate agonist, by blocking the NMDA receptor when it is active and thereby protecting the neuron without interfering with processes necessary for learning and memory (for a detailed review, see Sonkusare, Kaul, & Ramarao, 2005).

Regarding the effectiveness of NMDA, the efficacy of memantine has been demonstrated in randomized controlled trials (for a review of randomized control trials since 1991 see Möbius, 2003). In a review of research on memantine, Sonkusare, Kaul, & Ramarao (2005) conclude that memantine might be able to prevent further neurodegeneration in dementia of the Alzheimer's type. General information for memantine is available at www.namenda.com.

Psychoptropic Medication for Challenging Behaviors. The U.S. FDA has not approved the use of any psychotropic medication for the treatment of any challenging behaviors in persons with dementia (Profenno & Tariot, 2004, but also see Lawlor, 2004). In 2005 the FDA advised against the use

---

*Merz, the patent holder for memantine, withdrew Akatinol® from the market on July 31, 2002, and reintroduced the identical substance one day later as Axura®. The name change and the new label indication for moderate to severe dementia were accompanied by a 74% increase in price (Schmitt-Feuerbach, 2002). Merz entered strategic licensing and cooperation agreements with Lundbeck (Denmark) and Forest Laboratories (U.S.). The U.S. Food and Drug Administration approved Nemantin® in 2003. Memantine is now marketed worldwide as Axura® (Merz), Ebixa® (Lundbeck), and Nemantin® (Forest Laboratories).

of atypical antipsychotics for behavior problems occurring in dementia due to increased risk of death. Psychotropic medication should be used only after a thorough assessment to rule out medical conditions that might be causing or contributing to the problem behavior (e.g., infection, delirium, conditions causing pain). Nonpharmacological management of behavioral problems is the first-line approach. Psychotropic medications should be considered only after behavioral interventions have failed, or in case of an emergency (see Fisher, Cardinal, Yury, & Buchanan, in press, for guidelines on the pharmacological treatment of behavior problems in dementia).

Psychological Treatments

Given that there is currently no treatment available for halting or reversing the deterioration in degenerative forms of dementia, treatment planning for persons with dementia should focus on maintaining the patient's repertoire for as long as possible and preventing or reducing *excess* disability (Fisher, in press). In the context of a degenerative dementia, excess disability can be conceptualized as a premature reduction in behaviors that will inevitably be lost due to the disease process (Fisher, in press). For example, persons with Alzheimer's disease will eventually lose all verbal abilities; as the person's verbal abilities decline, alternative forms of communication may emerge (e.g., repeating the same question in order to access social attention or repeatedly calling the same name in order to access sensory stimulation). Interventions to reduce disruptive vocalizations that suppress functionally important vocal behavior may ultimately contribute to excess disability by causing a premature reduction in verbal behavior (Fisher, in press; Ritchie, Touchon, & Ledesert, 1998).

Managing Emotional Problems in Dementia. Cognitive behavior therapy is effective for the treatment of depression in mildly impaired persons with dementia (Gallagher-Thompson et al., 2000). Activity programs and interventions based on a behavioral activation model have also been found to be effective in reducing depression and improving affect in elderly persons with dementia (Teri et al., 1999). Relaxation-based interventions have been found to be effective for reducing anxiety in older adults with dementia.

Managing Behavioral Problems. Behavioral problems such as aggression, wandering, repeated questions, and public displays of sexual behavior are leading risk factors for institutionalization in persons with dementia (Hope, Keene, Gedling, Fairburn, & Jacoby, 1998). More than 50% of patients developing behaviors warrant intervention (Chen, Borson, & Scanlan, 2000).

Behavioral interventions are effective for reducing and preventing behavior problems in dementia because they are highly influenced by environmental stimuli, even in advanced dementia (Buchanan & Fisher, 2002; Burgio et al., 1994; Fisher, in press). Recent data suggest that problem behaviors that occur in degenerative dementia are adaptive in that they reliably occur in the context of specific antecedent stimuli (e.g., conditions of high or low stimulation) and are consistently followed by specific consequences (e.g., attention or the removal of an aversive stimulus). These findings suggest that the so-called problem behaviors serve important adaptive functions for patients. Given the fragility of the behavioral repertoires of persons with dementia, these behaviors should be treated with great care as they may be the only behaviors available for serving important functions such as accessing attention, communicating distress, or accessing sensory stimulation. Interventions for behavior problems should be designed to address the function of the problem behavior (Fisher, in press) and not solely focused on its reduction or elimination.

Interventions to Enhance Caregiver Functioning

Caregivers of persons with dementia are at very high risk for negative outcomes. Research since the mid-1980s has consistently found that emotional coping and instrumental skill repertoires have a large influence on the caregiving experience. The emotional quality of the premorbid relationship (e.g., whether the caregiver felt affection for or disliked the person with dementia) can also influence the caregiver's emotional experience and willingness to accept the burden of providing care. Given the heterogeneity of emotional coping, instrumental skills, problems-solving skills, and relationship histories across caregiver/patient dyads, providers should develop individualized support plans based on the caregiver/patient dyad's specific needs. Four domains relevant for effective caregiver functioning should be assessed:

1. *Knowledge of effects of dementia* and how it affects the patient's behavior (e.g., does the caregiver interpret patient's behavior to be intentional or due to the disease?).
2. *Emotion regulation and problem-solving skills* for managing common emotional stressors associated with caregiving (e.g., sleep deprivation, patient's resistance to care).

3. *Skill repertoire for managing instrumental tasks* associated with caregiving (e.g., does the caregiver have experience as a parent or grandparent in bathing, feeding, managing medication for another person; are his or her communication and assertion skills effective for their role as a patient advocate?).
4. *Relationship quality* (how does the caregiver/patient dyad's relationship history affect the emotional response of the caregiver to the patient?).

Measures. Measures designed for the assessment of specific problems in the general population (e.g., measures of anxiety, depression, substance use, sleep disturbance) may be helpful in treatment planning and should be selected based on an individual caregiver's presentation. Measures designed specifically for assessing problems associated with caregiving include those listed in Table 6.1.

What Are Effective Treatments for Caregivers? A meta-analysis of interventions for family caregivers (Sorensen, Pinquart, & Duberstein, 2002) and reviews of the dementia caregiver intervention literature (e.g., Schulz et al., 2002; Steffen & Mangum, in press) indicate that psychoeducational interventions have a greater effect on caregiver outcomes (e.g., knowledge, burden, depression) compared to more traditional support group formats. In particular, psychoeducational interventions using behavioral and cognitive

TABLE 6.1   Instruments for Problems Associated with Caregiving

Instrument	Length (items)	Specific Purposes
Caregiver Task Checklist (Gallagher-Thompson et al., 2000)	29	Assess basic and instrumental activities for which assistance is provided (e.g., grooming, toileting, meals, transportation, bathing, and finances) and whether the caregiver finds the task difficult, tiring, or upsetting to perform.
Revised Memory and Behavior Problem	24	Assess frequency and caregiver burden associated with patient's memory-related problems, disruptive behaviors, and depression.
The Revised-Ways of Coping Checklist (RWCCL) (Vitaliano, Russo, Carr, Maiuro, & Becker, 1985)	41	Assess emotional coping strategies (e.g., problem solving, support focused, avoidance, and blaming self) in caregivers of persons with dementia.

treatment strategies have been found to have the greatest impact on caregiver depressive symptoms and other indexes of psychological health. These interventions tend to be structured and time limited, employing guided mastery to teach behavioral, emotional, and cognitive self-regulation skills through direct instruction, in-session practice, and between-session assignments.

Effective interventions include:

- *Coping With Caregiving,* a cognitive behavioral intervention designed to teach skills including relaxation, perspective taking, and goal setting for managing mood (Coon, Thompson, Steffen, Sorocco, & Gallagher-Thompson, 2003; Gallagher-Thompson et al., 2003).
- *Coping With Frustration,* a cognitive behavioral intervention for the treatment of anger and frustration related to caregiving. Components include relaxation training, techniques for challenging dysfunctional thoughts, and assertion training (Gallagher-Thompson, & DeVries, 1994; Steffen, 2000).
- Training in coping with challenging behaviors. Training and intervention packages are available for increasing caregivers' ability to manage behavior problems of the person receiving care and for improving problem-solving skills (e.g., Burgio, Stevens, Guy, Roth, & Haley, in press). Support for specific problems (e.g., sleep disturbance in the patient or caregiver, incontinence, home safety, problem solving regarding extended care options, issues regarding legal guardianship, end of life care) can be provided in group format (e.g., in the form of caregiver classes) or on an individual basis as needed.

Information regarding evidence-based care of persons with dementia is available through the following resources:

- Alzheimer's Disease Education and Referral (ADEAR) Center 1-800-438-4380, 301-495-3334 (fax); Web address: http://www.alzheimers.org. This service of the National Institute on Aging is funded by the federal government. It offers information and publications on diagnosis, treatment, patient care, caregiver needs, long-term care, education and training, and research related to Alzheimer's disease. Staff answer telephone and written requests and make referrals to local and national resources. Publications and videos can be ordered through the ADEAR Center or via the Web site.
- Alzheimer's Association, 1-800-272-3900; Web address: http://www.alz.org.

- Eldercare Locator. Information regarding case management resources for elderly persons with dementia is available at 1-800-677-1116; Web address: http://www.eldercare.gov. The Eldercare Locator is a nationwide, directory assistance service helping older people and their caregivers locate local support and resources for older Americans. It is funded by the Administration on Aging (AoA).

SCHIZOPHRENIA IN LATE LIFE

Basic Facts About Schizophrenia

Schizophrenia is a chronic psychiatric disorder that severely disrupts cognitive, emotional, and behavioral functioning (American Psychiatric Association, 1994, p. 274). It is best characterized as a heterogeneous disorder, as no essential symptom must be present for diagnosis. Accordingly, there are numerous paths by which individuals meet diagnostic criteria.

Schizophrenia is among the most debilitating of psychiatric illnesses. It has a lifetime prevalence of 1% in all countries and affects all ethnic groups (Walker, Kestler, Bollini, & Hochman, 2004). The prevalence in elderly persons living in the community is less than 1% (Merck, 2000). It is estimated that between 3.2% and 10% of elderly patients in psychiatric facilities have schizophrenia (Karon & VandenBos, 1998).

Symptoms are generally dichotomized into positive and negative symptom clusters (Bradford, Stroup, & Lieberman, 2002). Positive symptoms include delusions, hallucinations, and disorganized thinking (i.e., formal thought disorder). Positive symptoms arise outside the realm of normal experience. For example, a person might see or hear things that are not externally verifiable (e.g., no one else sees the visual phenomenon). Negative symptoms include affective flattening, alogia (e.g., restriction in the amount of spontaneous speech), avolution (i.e., problems initiating goal-directed activities), and anhedonia (i.e., lack of pleasure) (American Psychiatric Association, 1994, pp. 276, 764). Negative symptoms suggest that there is something missing from the individual's experience. For example, while most people become elated after finding $100 in the street, persons experiencing negative symptoms (particularly anhedonia) may show no emotional reaction whatsoever.

The *DSM-IV* denotes five subtypes of schizophrenia: Paranoid Type, Disorganized Type, Catatonic Type, Undifferentiated Type, and Residual Type (American Psychiatric Association, 1994). The essential feature of the *Paranoid Type* is a preponderance of delusions or hallucinations, all the while cognitive functioning and affect remain relatively intact. The essential features of the *Disorganized Type* are "disorganized speech, disorganized behavior, and flat or inappropriate affect" (American Psychiatric Association, 1994, pp. 287–288). This subtype typically runs an unremitting course. The essential feature of the *Catatonic Type* is a considerable psychomotor disturbance, such as catalepsy (i.e., limbs are suspended in a fixed position), excess motoric activity, and echolalia (i.e., pathologically echoing what others say). The *Undifferentiated Type* "is the presence of symptoms that meet Criterion A of schizophrenia but that do not meet criteria for the Paranoid, Disorganized, or Catatonic Type" (p. 289). The *Residual Type*, therefore, is characterized by at least one episode of schizophrenia, in which the individual continues to experience negative symptoms in the absence of positive psychotic symptoms.

Older persons who meet the diagnostic criteria for schizophrenia fall into one of two categories: individuals who developed schizophrenia earlier in life and still present with symptoms (early-onset schizophrenia), and those who develop schizophrenia for the first time in middle to old age (i.e., after 45 years of age, late-onset schizophrenia or paraphrenia; Rodriguez-Ferrera, Vassilas, & Haque, 2004; Bartels, Mueser, & Miles, 1998).

Cohort differences in treatment history have had a significant impact on the lives of elderly persons with schizophrenia who were hospitalized prior to and after the advent of antipsychotic medications. As the majority of typical antipsychotics were introduced between 1954 and 1975, patients who were hospitalized in psychiatric settings prior to the mid-1950s, were commonly prescribed psychosurgery, which entails the ablation of parts of the frontal lobes (there were 10,000 such operations in the United States by August 1949; Jansson, 2005), electroconvulsive therapy, and insulin shock therapy in efforts at managing difficult behaviors (Moniz, 1962; Sakel, 1938; Shen, 1999). Given this history with the health-care community, many patients, having been exposed to these highly invasive interventions, may believe that such practices still take place in their current residence (e.g., skilled nursing facility). The advent of antipsychotic medications not only heralded a rapid decline in the use of psychosurgery, electroconvulsive therapy, and insulin shock therapy, it also sparked rapid deinstitutionalization from psychiatric hospitals to community mental health settings (Krupinski, 1995). It is estimated that between 1955 and 1980 the number of patients residing in psychiatric hospitals dropped precipitously from 559,000 to 150,000 (Department of Health and Human Services, 1981). Although deinstitutionalization improved the lives of many persons with schizophrenia, for others this movement was largely a shift between institutions, namely, from psychiatric hospitals to nursing homes (Meeks et al., 1990). About 50% of patients with schizophrenia made such a transition (Schmidt et al., 1977). This cohort, therefore, lived very little of their adult lives outside of an institution. Accordingly, this institutional history would place limits on what might be expected as far as their independence is concerned (e.g., assisted living might be too hard of a transition for some).

Regarding treatment history, symptoms, and stability, older adults with schizophrenia tend to be highly heterogeneous (e.g., length of time spent in hospitals; duration of treatment with neuroleptic drugs) (Meeks et al., 1990). Meeks and colleagues showed that, while long periods of stability were common, complete absence of symptoms was rare. This disorder generally adheres to the "law of thirds" (Kopelowicz, Lieberman, & Zarate, 2002). About a third of individuals return to premorbid functioning following one or more psychotic episodes. Another third have many years of recurrent acute psychotic episodes, with periods of full or partial remission. The final third experience persistent psychotic symptoms without significant remissions. Elderly persons with schizophrenia have a global recovery rate of about 21% (Meeks et al., 1990). Suicide is the leading cause of death in persons with schizophrenia (Schwartz & Cohen, 2001); approximately 10% commit suicide (American Psychiatric Association, 1994). While suicide has received much attention in younger persons with schizophrenia, there is a dearth in the literature with respect to older adults. One study that examined computerized admission records ($N = 1066$) of 692 patients with schizophrenia over 60 years of age suggested that 4.6% of admissions were due to suicide attempts (Barak, Knobler, & Aizenberg, 2004).

Regarding etiology, it is widely accepted that schizophrenia results from interacting biological and environmental causes (Meeks, 2000). That is, an individual might have a genetic or biological predisposition toward schizophrenia (e.g., a parent has schizophrenia or the person has certain brain anomalies that are correlated with the disorder). Highly stressful environments (e.g., constant fighting in the home) can thus trigger the disease in those individuals with biological susceptibilities. By contrast, other individuals, lacking this biological disposition, probably would not develop schizophrenia under similar circumstances. Treatment, therefore, would consist of either (1) reducing biological vulnerability (e.g., corrective medication), (2) reducing environmental stressors, or (3) teaching patients how to better cope with their life circumstances (Bartels, Mueser, & Miles, 1998).

Assessment

What Is Involved in Effective Assessment?

The diagnosis of schizophrenia should be made only after a thorough medical workup. Once medical conditions are ruled out, a comprehensive assessment of schizophrenia should include an examination of *DSM* criteria for schizophrenia, functional impairment, psychiatric history, family history of psychiatric illness, psychiatric comorbidity, substance use, and suicide risk.

Patients often rate themselves as significantly healthier in regard to social impairment, symptoms, and global functioning compared to clinicians' ratings (McGlashan, 1984). Ideally, a comprehensive assessment includes both clinician and self-report indexes (see Table 6.2). Readers should note

TABLE 6.2   Instruments for Assessing Schizophrenia

Instrument	Description/Characteristics
Clinician-Administered Measures	
The Structured Clinical Interview for DSM-IV Axis I Disorders (SCID-I) (First, Spitzer, Gibbon, & Williams, 1996)	Can guide clinicians through the differential diagnosis process, ruling in and ruling out major diagnostic categories.
Global Assessment of Functioning (GAF) Scale (American Psychiatric Association, 1994)	A global rating of overall psychological, social, and occupational functioning, ranging from 0 to 100, with 100 suggesting "superior functioning in a wide range of activities" and 10 suggesting "persistent danger of severely hurting self or others."
	Limited information about the patient.
Self-Report Measures	
The Subjective Well-being Under Neuroleptics Scale (Naber, 1995)	Assess the subjective impact of treatment on patients' quality of life.
	Track subjective changes (e.g., restrictions in emotions and clarity of thinking).
	Useful in identifying adverse drug reactions.
The Medication Event Monitoring System (MEMS) (Diaz et al., 2001)	89% of patients with schizophrenia fail to take their medication as prescribed (Lacro, Dunn, Dolder, Leckband, & Jeste, 2002).
	Nonadherence can have a profound impact on functioning and quality of life.
	A reliable means of assessing adherence, with a computer chip built into the bottle cap to record the time and date each time the cap is opened.
	The downside to this device is its cost.
The Medication Adherence Rating Scale (MARS) (Thompson, Kularni, & Sergejew, 2000)	A 10-item, paper-and-pencil, self-report scale, valid and reliable.
	An inexpensive alternative to the MEMS.
	Medication adherence monitoring is achieved in one of three ways: laboratory tests (e.g., urinalysis), pill counts, and self-report.
Experience of Caregiving Inventory (Szmukler et al., 1996)	A 66-item questionnaire assessing the negative and positive impact of the patient's illness on his or her caregiver(s).

that the use of these measures have not been tested with elderly persons with schizophrenia.

The clinician-administered measures are useful in making a diagnosis and in determining the general level of impairment, particularly when assessing community-dwelling elderly persons who, to a large extent, live independently. The first three self-report measures are helpful in assessing medication-related factors as they pertain to treatment adherence. The last self-report measure concerns family caregivers. Most community-dwelling elderly persons with schizophrenia rely heavily on family in activities of daily living, treatment coordination, and the like (Meeks et al., 1990).

What Assessments Are Not Helpful?

Projective tests, such as the Rorshach and Thematic Apperception Test (TAT) should not be used in assessing schizophrenia as they are not valid.

Evidence-Based Interventions for Schizophrenia

Schizophrenia is best treated from a biopsychosocial perspective, involving a multidisciplinary treatment team (Bartels, Mueser, & Miles, 1998). The biopsychosocial model considers biological, psychological, and social variables in assessment and treatment.

What Is Effective Medical Treatment?

Antipsychotic medication is typically the first line of treatment in managing the acute psychotic phase of the disorder and residual symptoms (Bradford, Stroup, & Lieberman, 2002). The newer atypical antipsychotic drugs (e.g., clozapine, risperidone, olanzapine) are recommended over conventional antipsychotic medications (e.g., haloperidol, thioridazine) for elderly populations because they produce fewer adverse effects (Conley, 2000; Merck, 2000). Fewer side effects notwithstanding, the use of any antipsychotic medication can be potentially dangerous in elderly patients, as elderly persons experience two to three times the rate of adverse drug reactions compared to younger persons due to multimorbidity, polypharmacy, and age-related changes in pharmacokinetic and pharmacodynamic characteristics (Turnheim, 1998, 2004). Anticholinergic reactions, tardive dyskinesia (persistent involuntary movements), sedation, and orthostatic hypotension (sudden drop in blood pressure when changing positions) are several side effects of particular concern in elderly populations because they can lead to serious falls and accidents (Arana, 2000; Masand, 2000, p. 43).

To reduce the risk of drug interactions and noncompliance, drug regimens should be structured as simply as possible (i.e., one or two treatments daily; Turnheim, 2004). Moreover, in light of an increased risk of side effects, lower doses are almost always recommended (Castle & Howard, 1992). For example, initial daily doses should not exceed 1 mg of risperidone and 5 mg of olanzapine (Merck, 2000, p. 332). Additional risk factors affecting dosage include gender (due to lower body mass, women are at greater risk), tobacco use, comorbid illness (e.g., Alzheimer's disease), and hepatic or renal impairment (Madhusoodanan, Sinha, Brenner, Gupta, & Bogunovic, 2001, p. 210).

There is only a scant amount of data on the pharmacological treatment of schizophrenia in the elderly (Bartels, Mueser, & Miles, 1998). While the available evidence suggests that antipsychotic medication can prove beneficial in elderly populations, the effect sizes are modest at best, and medications are seldom sufficient in and of themselves (Meeks, 2000). Invariably, psychosocial interventions are also necessary.

What Are Effective Psychosocial Treatments?

Most surveys suggest that between 25% and 50% of patients continue to experience significant psychotic symptoms, in spite of optimal pharmacotherapy (Gould, Mueser, Bolton, Mays, & Goff, 2001). Moreover, it is estimated that over a third of patients with schizophrenia experience medication-resistant symptoms (Garety, Fowler, & Kuipers, 2000). Accordingly, psychosocial therapies are critical in the management of schizophrenia. However, with respect to elderly persons with schizophrenia, the optimal psychosocial interventions have yet to be determined. In a recent meta-analytic review of psychosocial programs for schizophrenia in younger adults, cognitive therapy, cognitive behavioral therapy, and social skills training (including social problem solving) all reported positive findings (Bustillo, Lauriello, Horan, & Keith, 2001).

Cognitive Therapy and Cognitive Behavioral Therapy. Cognitive and cognitive behavioral intervention approaches directly modify specific thoughts or beliefs that supposedly mediate maladaptive behavioral and emotional responding (Beck, 1976; Ellis, 1962; 1971). The goals of these treatments are to reduce the conviction of delusional thoughts, thus affecting severity, and, alternatively, promoting more effective coping strategies (Gould, Mueser, Bolton, Mays, & Goff, 2001).

Social Skills Training. Social skills training involves teaching patients effective interpersonal behavior (e.g., how to make a request assertively).

Although the impact of social skills training on symptoms remains unclear, "it remains an important avenue for improving social functioning" (Bartels, Mueser, & Miles, 1998, p. 186).

While these techniques are promising, caution is in order, because these effects tend to be domain-specific and do not necessarily result in improvements in other areas (Bustillo, Lauriello, Horan, & Keith, 2001). Moreover, these findings have not been adequately evaluated in older persons.

What Are Effective Self-Help Treatments?

There are dozens of self-help books on the market today. Of the two listed here, neither has been empirically validated, independently, or as part of a treatment package. However, the advice provided is in accordance with empirically based treatment.

- *Surviving schizophrenia: A manual for families, consumers, and providers,* by E. F. Torrey (2001).
- *Coping with schizophrenia: A guide for families,* by K. T. Mueser and S. Gingerich (1994).

Here are some useful Web sites:

- http://www.nlm.nih.gov/medlineplus/schizophrenia.html
- http://www.schizophrenia.com/
- http://my.webmd.com/hw/schizophrenia/aa47138.asp?z=1835_00000_0000_rl_08
- http://members.aol.com/leonardjk/USA.htm (schizophrenia support organizations)
- http://www.nami.org/Template.cfm?Section=By_Illness&template=/ContentManagement/ContentDisplay.cfm&ContentID=7416
- http://www.rcpsych.ac.uk/info/help/schiz/Schizophrenia.pdf
- http://www.mentalhealth.org/publications/allpubs/ken98-0052/default.asp
- http://www.mentalhealth.org/publications/allpubs/ken98-0050/default.asp (how to pay for mental health services)

How Does One Select Among Treatments?

Patients should be well informed about the extant evidence-based treatment options available, including psychological and medical interventions. Should clinicians elect to use medication treatment, possible side effects and drug interactions should be discussed with patients or their guardians. Other issues to consider are comparative treatment expenses, suicide risk, environmental support (e.g., is the patient homeless?), and previous treatment successes and failures.

Other Issues in the Treatment and Management of Schizophrenia

Drug Holidays. Some elderly may no longer require antipsychotic medication. Try periodic trials of discontinuation, under careful supervision (Merck, 2000).

Relapse/Suicide Prevention. The likelihood of suicide and relapse is greatest within the first 14 weeks following discharge (Maxmen & Ward, 1994). Caton (1984) recommends the following, when discharge planning, to help mitigate against suicide and relapse: (1) provide patient and family education about the purpose and importance of taking medication as prescribed; (2) prepare patients for aftercare by walking them through the logistics of making outpatient appointments, obtaining transportation, and the like; (3) provide patients with adequate case management (to help them find housing and financial support); (4) facilitate patient connection with community organizations (e.g., volunteer services and leisure activities) to help maintain social skills; and (5) conduct psychoeducation for the family about the disease and how to better express themselves emotionally around the patient (e.g., anger management).

REFERENCE AND RESOURCE LIST

AD 2000 Collaborative Group. (2004). Long-term donepezil treatment in 565 patients with Alzheimer's disease (AD 2000): Randomised double-blind trial. *Lancet, 363,* 2105–2115.

American Psychiatric Association. (1994). *Diagnostic and statistical manual of mental disorders* (4th ed.). Washington, DC: Author.

Arana, G. W. (2000). An overview of side effects caused by typical antipsychotics. *Journal of Clinical Psychiatry, 61,* 5–11.

Barak, Y., Knobler, C. Y., & Aizenberg, D. (2004). Suicide attempts amongst elderly schizophrenia patients: A 10-year case-control study. *Schizophrenia Research, 71,* 77–81.

Bartels, S. J., Mueser, K. T., & Miles, K. M. (1998). Schizophrenia. In M. Hersen & V. B. Van Hasselt (Eds.), *Handbook of clinical geropsychology* (pp. 173–194). New York: Plenum Press.

Beck, A. T. (1976). *Cognitive therapy and the emotional disorders.* New York: International Universities Press.

Bloom, M., Fischer, J., & Orme, J. G. (1995). *Evaluating practice: Guidelines for the accountable professional* (2nd ed.). Boston: Allyn and Bacon.

Bradford, D., Stroup, S., & Lieberman, J. (2002). Pharmacological treatments for schizophrenia. In P. E. Nathan & J. M. Gorman (Eds.), *A guide to treatments that work* (2nd ed. pp. 169–200). New York: Oxford University Press.

Buchanan, J. A., & Fisher, J. E. (2002). Noncontingent reinforcement as an intervention for disruptive vocalizations in Alzheimer's disease patients. *Journal of Applied Behavior Analysis, 35,* 99–103.

Burgio, L. D., Scilly, K., Hardin, J. M., Jankosky, J., Bonino, P., Slater, S. C., et al. (1994). Studying disruptive vocalization and contextual factors in the nursing home using computer-assisted real-time observation. *Journal of Gerontology: Psychological Sciences, 49,* P230–P239.

Burgio, L. D., & Stevens, A. B. (1999). Behavioral interventions and motivational systems in the nursing home. In R. Schultz, G. Maddox, & M. P. Lawton (Eds.), *Annual review of gerontology and geriatrics* (pp. 284–320). New York: Springer Publishing.

Burgio, L., Stevens, A., Guy, D., Roth, D. L., & Haley, W. E. (in press). Impact of two psychosocial interventions on White and African American family caregivers of individuals with dementia. *Gerontologist.*

Bustillo, J. R., Lauriello, J., Horan, W. P., & Keith, S. J. (2001). The psychosocial treatment of schizophrenia: An update. *American Journal of Psychiatry, 158,* 163–175.

Castle, D. J., & Howard, R. (1992). What do we know about the aetiology of late-onset schizophrenia? *European Psychiatry, 7,* 99–108.

Caton, C. L. M. (1984). *Management of chronic schizophrenia.* New York: Oxford University Press.

Centers for Disease Control and Prevention. (1999). Mortality from Alzheimer's disease: An update. *National Vital Statistics Reports, 47*(20).

Chen, J. C., Borson, S., & Scanlan, J. M. (2000). Stage-specific prevalence of behavioral symptoms in Alzheimer's disease in a multi-ethnic community sample. *American Journal of Geriatric Psychiatry, 8*(2), 123–133.

Cohen-Mansfield J., & Billig, N. (1986). Agitated behavior in the elderly: A conceptual review. *Journal of the American Geriatrics Society, 34,* 711–721.

Conley, R. R. (2000). Risperidone side effects. *Journal of Clinical Psychiatry, 61,* 20–23.

Coon, D. W., Thompson, L., Steffen, A., Sorocco, K., Gallagher-Thompson, D. (2003). Anger and depression management: Psychoeducational skills training interventions for women caregivers of a relative with dementia. *Gerontologist, 43*(5), 678–689.

Cummings, J. L. (2004). Alzheimer's disease. *New England Journal of Medicine, 351,* 56–67.

Department of Health and Human Services. (1981). *Towards a national plan for the chronically mentally ill.* Washington, DC: U.S. Government Printing Office.

Diaz, E., Levine, H. B., Sullivan, M. C., Sernyak, M. J., Hawkins, K. A., Cramer, J. A., et al. (2001). Use of the Medication Event Monitoring System to estimate medication compliance in patients with schizophrenia. *Journal of Psychiatry Neuroscience, 26,* 325–329.

Durand, M. V. & Crimmins, D. B. (1988). Identifying the variables maintaining self-injurious behavior. *Journal of Autism and Developmental Disorders, 18,* 88–117.

Ellis, A. (1962). *Reason and emotion in psychotherapy.* New York: Lyle Stuart.

Ellis, A. (1971). *Growth through reason.* North Hollywood, CA: Wilshire.

Evans, D. A., Funkenstein, H. H., Albert, M. S., Scherr, P. A., Cook, N. R., Chown, M. J., et al. (1989). Prevalence of Alzheimer's disease in a community population of older persons: Higher than previously reported, *Journal of the American Medical Association 262,* 2551.

First, M. B., Spitzer, R. L., Gibbon, M., & Williams, J. B. W. (1996). *Structured Clinical Interview for DSM-IV Axis I Disorders—Patient Edition* (SCID-I/P, Version 2.0). NY: Biometrics Research Department, New York State Psychiatric Institute.

Fisher, J. E. (in press). Promoting adaptive behavior in elderly persons with dementia. *Clinical Gerontologist.*

Fisher, J. E., Cardinal, C., Yury, C., & Buchanan, J. (in press). Dementia. In J. E. Fisher and W. O'Donohue (Eds.), *Practice guidelines for evidence-based psychotherapy.* New York: Springer Publishing.

Forsell, Y., & Wingblad, B. (1998). Major depression in a population of demented and nondemented older people: Prevalence and correlates. *Journal of the American Geriatrics Society, 46,* 27–30.

Gallagher-Thompson, D., & DeVries, H. (1994). "Coping with Frustration" classes: Development and preliminary outcomes with women who care for relatives with dementia. *Gerontologist, 34,* 548–552.

Gallagher-Thompson, D., Haley, W. E., Guy, D., Rubert, M., Arguelles, T., Tennstedt, et al. (2003). Tailoring psychosocial interventions for ethnically diverse dementia caregivers. *Clinical Psychology: Science and Practice, 10,* 423–438.

Gallagher-Thompson, D., Lovett, S., Rose, J., McKibbin, C., Coon, D., Futterman, A., et al. (2000). Impact of psychoeducational interventions on distressed family caregivers. *Journal of Clinical Geropsychology, 6,* 91–110.

Garety, P. A., Fowler, D., & Kuipers, E. (2000). Cognitive-behavioral therapy for medication resistant symptoms. *Schizophrenia Bulletin, 26,* 73–86.

Gould, R. A., Mueser, K. T., Bolton, E., Mays, V., & Goff, D. (2001). Cognitive therapy for psychosis in schizophrenia: An effect size analysis. *Schizophrenia Research, 48,* 335–342.

Gray, S. L., Lai, K. V., & Larson, E. B. (1999). Drug-induced cognition disorders in the elderly. *Drug Safety, 21*(2), 101–122.

Hope, T., Keene, J., Gedling, K., Fairburn, C. G., & Jacoby, R. (1998). Predictors of institutionalization for people with dementia living at home with a career. *International Journal of Geriatric Psychiatry 13*(10), 682–690.

Iwata, B. A. (1995). *Functional Analysis Screening Tool (FAST).* Florida Center on Self-Injury, University of Florida.

Jansson, B. (2005). *Controversial psychosurgery resulted in a Nobel Prize.* Retrieved June 14, 2005 from http://nobelprize.org/medicine/articles/moniz/.

Jones, R. W. (2003). Have cholinergic therapies reached their clinical boundary in Alzheimer's disease. *International Journal of Geriatric Psychiatry, 18,* S7–S13.

Kaduzkiewicz, H., Beck-Bornholdt, H. P., van den Bussche, H., & Zimmermann, T. (2004). Fragliche Evidenz fuer den Einsatz des Cholinesterasehemmers Donepezil bei Alzheimer-Demenz—eine systematische Uebersichtsarbeit. *Fortschritte der Neurologischen Psychiatrie, 72*(10), 557–563.

Karon, B. P., & VandenBos, G. R. (1998). Schizophrenia and psychosis in elderly populations. In I. H. Nordhus, G. R. VandenBos, S. Berg & P. Fromholt (Eds.), *Clinical geropsychology* (pp. 219–227). Washington, DC: American Psychological Association.

Kopelowicz, A., Liberman, R. P., & Zarate, R. (2002). Psychosocial treatments for schizophrenia. In P. E. Nathan & J. M. Gorman (Eds.), *A guide to treatments that work* (2nd ed., pp. 201–228). New York: Oxford University Press.

Krupinski, J. (1995). De-institutionalization of psychiatric patients: Progress or abandonment? *Social Sciences Medicine, 40,* 577–579.

Lacro, J. P., Dunn, L. B., Dolder, C. R., Leckband, S. G., & Jeste, D. V. (2002). Prevalence of and risk factors for medication nonadherence in patients with schizophrenia: A comprehensive review of the literature. *Journal of Clinical Psychiatry, 63,* 892–909.

Lawlor, B. A. (2004). Behavioral and psychological symptoms in dementia: The role of atypical antipsychotics. *Journal of Clinical Psychiatry, 65*(11), S5–S10.

Lerman, D. C., & Iwata, B. A. (1993). Descriptive and experimental analyses of variables maintaining self-injurious behavior. *Journal of Applied Behavior Analysis, 26,* 293–319.

Madhusoodanan, S., Sinha, S., Brenner, R., Gupta, S., & Bogunovic, O. (2001). Use of olanzapine for elderly patients with psychotic disorders: A review. *Annals of Clinical Psychiatry, 13,* 201–213.

Masand, P. S. (2000). Side effects of antipsychotics in the elderly. *Journal of Clinical Psychiatry, 61,* 43–49.

Maxmen, J. S., & Ward, N. G. (1994). *Essential psychopathology and its treatment* (2nd ed.). New York: W. W. Norton & Company.

McGlashan, T. H. (1984). The Chestnut Lodge follow-up study: II. Long-term outcome of schizophrenia and the affective disorders. *Archives of General Psychiatry, 41,* 586–601.

Meeks, S. (2000). Schizophrenia and related disorders. In S. K. Whitbourne (Ed.), *Psychopathology in later adulthood* (pp. 189–215). New York: Wiley.

Meeks, S., Carstensen, L. L., Stafford, P. B., Brenner, L. L., Weathers, F., Welch, R., & Oltmanns, T. F. (1990). Mental health needs of the chronically mentally ill. *Psychology and Aging, 5,* 163–171.

Merck. (2000). *The Merck manual of geriatrics* (3rd ed.). White House Station, NJ: Merck Research Laboratories.

Möbius, H. J. (2003). Memantine: Update on the current evidence. *International Journal of Geriatric Psychiatry, 18,* S47–S54.

Moniz, E. (1962). *Tentatives opératoires dans traitement de certaines psychoses.* Paris: Masson.

Mueser, K. T., & Gingerich, S. (1994). *Coping with schizophrenia: A guide for families.* Oakland, CA: New Harbinger Publications.

Naber, D. (1995). A self-rating to measure subjective effects of neuroleptic drugs, relationships to objective psychopathology, quality of life, compliance and other clinical variables. *International Clinical Psychopharmacology, 10*(Suppl. 3), 133–138.

National Institute of Neurological Diseases and Stroke. (2005). Retrieved from http://www.ninds.gov.

National Institute on Aging. (2005). Alzheimer's Disease Education & Referral Center (ADEAR). Retrieved from http://www.alzheimers.org/causes.htm.

NIH Consensus Statement Online. (1987). *Differential Diagnosis of Dementing Diseases.* Jul [cited 11/13/2004]; 6(11):1–27. Retrieved from http://consensus.nih.gov/cons/063/063_statement.htm

Pinquart, M., & Sorenson, S. (2003). Differences between caregivers and noncaregivers in psychological health and physical health: A meta-analysis. *Psychology and Aging, 18*(2), 250–267.

Profenno, L. A., & Tariot, P. N. (2004). Pharmacologic management of agitation in Alzheimer's disease. *Dementia and Geriatric Cognitive Disorders, 17,* 65–77.

Ritchie, K., Touchon, J., & Ledesert, B. (1998). Progressive disability in senile dementia is accelerated in the presence of depression. *International Journal of Geriatric Psychiatry, 13,* 459–461.

Rodriguez-Ferrera, S., Vassilas, C. A., & Haque, S. (2004). Older people with schizophrenia: A community study in a rural catchment area. *International Journal of Geriatric Psychiatry, 19,* 1181–1187.

Sakel, M. (1938). The pharmacological shock treatment of schizophrenia. *Nervous and Mental Disease Monograph, 62.*

Schmitt-Feuerbach, B. (2002). Eine neue Karriere fuer den bewaehrten Wirkstoff Memantine. Aerzte Zeitung Online. Retrieved November 14, 2004, from http://www.aerztezeitung.de/docs/2002/11/04/198a1401.asp?cat=/medizin/alzheimer

Schneider, L. S. (2004). AD 2000: Donepezil in Alzheimer's disease. *Lancet, 363,* 2100–2101.

Schulz, R., O'Brien, A. T., Bookwala, J., & Fleissner, K. (1995). Psychiatric and physical morbidity effects of dementia caregiving: Prevalence, correlates, and causes. *Gerontologist, 36*(6), 771–791.

Schulz, R., O'Brien, A., Czaja, S., Ory, M., Norris, R., Martire, L. M., et al. (2002). Dementia caregiver intervention research: In search of clinical significance. *Gerontologist, 42*(5), 589.

Schwartz, R. C., & Cohen, B. N. (2001). Risk factors for suicidality among clients with schizophrenia. *Journal of Counseling and Development, 79,* 314–319.

Shen, W. W. (1999). A history of antipsychotic drug development. *Comprehensive Psychiatry, 40,* 407–414.

Sonkusare, S. K., Kaul, C. L., & Ramarao, P. (2005). Dementia of Alzheimer's disease and other neurodegenerative disorders—memantine, a new hope. *Pharmacological Research, 51,* 1–17.

Sorensen, S., Pinquart, M., & Duberstein, P. (2002). How affective are interventions with caregivers? An updated meta-analysis. *Gerontologist, 42*(3), 356–372.

Steffen, A. M. (2000). Anger management for dementia caregivers: A preliminary study using video and telephone interventions. *Behavior Therapy, 31,* 281–299.

Steffen, A. M., & Mangum, K. R. (in press). Reducing psychosocial distress in family caregivers: The case for behavioral and cognitive interventions. *Clinical Gerontology.*

Stewart, N., & Fairweather, S. (2002). Delirium: The physician's perspective. In R. Jacoby & C. Oppenheimer (Eds.), *Psychiatry in the elderly* (3rd ed., pp. 592–615). Oxford, UK: Oxford University Press.

Szmukler, G. I., Burgess, P., Herman, H., Benson, A., Colusa, S., & Bloch, S. (1996). Caring for relatives with serious mental illness: The development of the Experience of Caregiving Inventory. *Social Psychiatric Epistemology, 31,* 137–148.

Teri, L., et. al. (1999). Treatment of behavioral and mood disturbances in dementia. *Generations, 33,* 50–56.

Thompson, K., Kularni, J., & Sergejew, A. A. (2000). Reliability and validity of a new Medication Adherence Rating Scale (MARS) for the psychoses. *Schizophrenia Research, 42,* 241–247.

Torrey, E. F. (2001). *Surviving schizophrenia: A manual for families, consumers, and providers* (4th ed.). New York: Harper & Row, Publishers.

Turnheim, K. (1998). Drug dosage in the elderly. *Drugs Aging, 13,* 357–379.

Turnheim, K. (2004). Drug therapy in the elderly. *Experimental Gerontology, 39,* 1731–1738.

Vitaliano, P. P., Russo, J., Carr, J. E., Maiuro, R. D., & Becker, J. (1985). The ways of coping checklist: Revision and psychometric properties. *Multivariate Behavioral Research, 20,* 3–26.

Walker, E., Kestler, L., Bollini, A., & Hochman, K. M. (2004). Schizophrenia: Etiology and course. *Annual Review of Psychology, 55,* 401–430.

Zhang, L., Zhou, F., & Dani, J. A. (2004). Cholinergic drugs for Alzheimer's disease enhance in vitro dopamine release. *Molecular Pharmacology, 66*(3), 538–544.

CHAPTER 7

Evidence-Based Practices by Service Delivery Process

Jeffrey A. Buchanan and Tiffany Berg

In recent years, there has been considerable progress in identifying behavioral health interventions that demonstrate efficacy, resulting in products such as evidence-based practice (EBP) guidelines and the American Psychological Association's list of "empirically supported treatments" (Chambless et al., 1998). A number of evidence-based behavioral health practices are targeted specifically for older adults (Gatz et al., 1998).

Despite the fact that there are many well-established behavioral health interventions for older adults, one significant challenge is channeling these interventions to the older adults who will benefit from them. Many factors contribute to this impediment, including stigma associated with seeking mental health services, transportation difficulties, and the lack of clinicians with specialized training in working with older adults (Bartels, 2003). In addition, older adults are less likely to identify mental health needs or seek services (Mickus, Colenda, & Hogan, 2000). The goal of this chapter is to describe effective approaches for delivering EBPs to older adults. More specifically, it describes effective methods for screening and assessing patients and provides information on the delivery of evidence-based prevention and intervention programs. This chapter focuses on models of EBP delivery for which there is some empirical evidence that the model is effective with regard to outcomes that are important to consumers, health-care administrators, and public policy officials. Examples of these outcomes include penetration rates, measures of symptom severity, general health outcomes, measures of daily functioning, consumer satisfaction, primary health-care utilization rates (i.e., medical cost offset), and delayed utilization of more costly forms of care (e.g., long-term care).

SCREENING AND ASSESSMENT

Before providing evidence-based interventions, an adequate screening and assessment of the patient must be completed to determine specific behavioral health concerns and to identify the most likely effective intervention.

Screening

Screening individuals for behavioral health concerns is a critical component in any system that implements EBPs as it allows practitioners to identify those individuals who could benefit from evidence-based interventions. Given that older adults are unlikely to initially present to a behavioral health specialist, the responsibility of screening falls on primary care. This responsibility creates a significant challenge because many primary care providers do not feel comfortable in their ability to make mental health diagnoses, and time pressures leave them little time to conduct behavioral health screening (U.S. Department of Health and Human Services, 1999). Therefore, screening tools must be brief yet still accurately predict which patients are likely to meet diagnostic criteria for a disorder. To increase practicality, screening assessments can be mailed to patients or completed as part of routine annual exams (HMO Workgroup on Care Management, 2002). Some health-care systems (e.g., Veterans Affairs medical clinics) have trained administrative staff to administer screening devices while patients wait for appointments.

Bartels (2003) suggested that the current health-care system lacks adequate screening programs for identifying older adults with behavioral health concerns. Effective screening methods have, however, been developed for some of the most common psychological conditions affecting older adults. Most of these methods are used in large managed care organizations, but could certainly be implemented in other settings such as general primary care practices or long-term care. For depression, the most common screening question involves asking patients if they have often felt "sad or blue." This one question appears to have comparable predictive accuracy to lengthier screening devices such as the Geriatric Depression Scale (GDS; Yesavage et al., 1983). In addition, Whooley, Avins, Miranda, and Browner (1997) found that two questions ("During the past month have you often been bothered by feeling down, depressed, or hopeless?" and "During the past month, have you often been bothered by little interest or pleasure in doing things?") were as accurate as more extensive screening instruments.

Similar brief screens have been developed for dementia. For example, an affirmative answer to a single question, "During the past few months have you had increasing problems with severe memory loss?" may be able to identify a substantial number of cases of cognitive impairment (HMO Workgroup on Care Management, 2002). For detecting potential alcohol abuse problems, the CAGE screen is available (Ewing, 1984). The CAGE questions ask individuals about whether they have ever felt the need to *cut* down on drinking, have they ever felt *annoyed* by criticisms of drinking, have they had *guilty* feelings about drinking, and have they ever had to take a morning *eye-opener*. The CAGE screen has been used to detect potential alcohol abuse problems in older adults (Rabins et al., 2000).

Screens that involve just a few questions are ideal for primary care settings because they are brief, easily interpreted, and reasonably accurate. In systems in which electronic medical charts are available, automated reminders that prompt practitioners to conduct screens can be included to increase compliance with screening procedures. In addition, in systems in which behavioral and primary health care are not fully integrated, if a patient screens positive for a condition, electronic flagging systems can alert other practitioners, thereby increasing the probability of a referral to behavioral health.

In addition to administering screening questions or instruments, another option for identifying high-risk individuals involves the use of administrative data. Computerized databases can be used to track and flag individuals who have risk factors such as a previous diagnosis of depression, frequent utilization of primary care, or the presence of medical conditions that cause disability (heart disease, stroke, or Parkinson's disease). As an example, Kaiser Permanente, Colorado Region, uses this kind of data to identify members who have recently been widowed (HMO Workgroup on Care Management, 2002). Once identified, members are contacted (with their consent) by a volunteer who provides information about local grief support groups.

Assessment

After a positive screen, more thorough assessment is required. The goal of the assessment is to make a diagnosis, select problem behaviors, evaluate the severity of the condition, assess motivation for treatment, match clients to available EBP protocols, and track clinical progress. Assessment procedures must be thorough, yet efficient, particularly within integrated systems of care, and therefore knowledge concerning the best assessment instruments is vital. It is beyond the scope of this chapter to provide an exhaustive listing of available assessment instruments, but see Hayes, Barlow, and Nelson-Gray (1999) for a series of assessment strategies or guidelines that can help practitioners achieve two important goals: complete a time- and cost-efficient assessment and track clinical progress. The reader is also referred to Lichtenberg's *Handbook of Assessment in Clinical Gerontology* (1999) for more detailed information about screening and assessment instruments appropriate for a variety of mental health conditions that affect older adults.

Nomothetic versus Ideographic Assessment

The first assessment strategy involves balancing nomothetic and ideographic assessment procedures. A *nomothetic approach* is useful for *establishing that someone has a particular disorder* such as depression and determining the severity of the symptoms. A nomothetic assessment strategy involves comparing a given individual to a larger group. The goal is to make a diagnosis and measure the severity of symptom presentation against that of others in that same diagnostic group. One strength of nomothetic assessment instruments is that they have well-established psychometric properties and normative data; thus individual scores can be compared to scores of the normative group. The GDS (Yesavage et al., 1983) is a commonly used nomothetic instrument to assess severity of depression in older adults while the Structured Clinical Interview for the *DSM-IV* (First, Spitzer, Gibbon, & Williams, 1996) is a nomothetic instrument useful for making a diagnosis of depression.

An *ideographic assessment* strategy is designed to *assess the individual's unique symptom presentation* (i.e., how do they *differ* from those of the larger diagnostic group). Ideographic instruments are specifically tailored to an individual and his or her presenting problem; therefore, they may be more useful for treatment planning and be more sensitive to the effects of an intervention because their content reflects the unique presenting problems of the client. Ideographic assessment is more concerned with *why* an individual might be depressed (e.g., inactivity and social isolation, marital conflict) and what intervention might be most appropriate (e.g., increasing activity and socialization, improving martial communication).

Ultimately, a balance of nomothetic and ideographic strategies may be most appropriate. Nomothetic measures such as the GDS can be useful for tracking treatment progress. Nomothetic strategies may also be required depending on the type of setting in which one works (e.g., a managed care organization). Some nomothetic instruments such as the Minnesota Multiphasic Personality Inventory-2 (Butcher, Dahlstrom, Graham, Tellgen, &

Kaemmer, 1989) are not likely to be clinically useful given that they are lengthy and that developers of evidence-based psychotherapies have reported that they are rarely useful for treatment planning (O'Donohue, Buchanan, & Fisher, 2000). Ideographic strategies are far more useful, however, in determining what intervention(s) might be most useful for a given individual. For example, although cognitive behavioral therapy is an empirically supported intervention for depression in older adults, it does not directly address potentially important factors such as interpersonal conflict that could contribute to depressed mood.

Data Collection Guidelines

It is important to choose at least some measures that are psychometrically sound and that have been validated for use with older adults. It can be tempting to use instruments that have been well validated with younger adults, assuming that they will provide valid information about older adults. One concern, however, is that the presentation of some psychological conditions may differ in older adults. For instance, the Beck Depression Inventory (BDI; Beck, Ward, Mendelson, Mock, & Erbaugh, 1961) is the most widely used self-report measure of depression, but it includes several items that inquire about somatic symptoms. Older adults may experience a number of somatic symptoms that are related to either normal aging or medical conditions and not due to depression, resulting in inflated scores on the BDI.

It is also important to gather assessment data early in the course of contact with clients. This information can serve as baseline data by which to compare subsequent measurements. Repeated measurement of key target symptoms allows the clinician and client to track progress and make adjustments to the treatment plan, as necessary. EBPs are not always effective for particular individuals, so tracking progress is important to ensure that progress is occurring or as a basis to switch or adjust intervention strategies. Computerized data tracking systems that administer, score, and graph data can reduce the amount of practitioner time that is devoted to repeated assessment, produce instant feedback concerning patient progress, and allow other practitioners to have access to outcome data. Monitoring treatment progress is also important for the larger system in which a practitioner works in order to substantiate continued provision of behavioral healthcare services.

When possible, practitioners should administer multiple measures for each target behavior. There is often no one true measure for a particular problem (Hayes, Barlow, & Nelson-Gray, 1999); therefore gathering multiple measures will increase the chances of detecting a treatment effect if one is present. When measuring a number of outcomes, it is recommended that more convenient measures be used more frequently, while more time-consuming measures be used less frequently. In addition, practitioners should gather information from multiple sources (e.g., spouses, physicians) to protect against biases that are associated with self-report.

Outcomes beyond changes in presenting symptoms should be measured and tracked whenever possible. For example, measuring constructs such as quality of life, daily functioning, and perceived ability to cope can determine if behavioral health interventions are having a broader impact on patient functioning beyond symptom reduction. At an even broader level of assessment, health-care systems are increasingly concerned with other outcomes such as utilization of primary care services, emergency room visits, prescription refills, and number of hospitalizations. Computerized client tracking systems can track these outcomes and data can be examined to evaluate whether those who utilize behavioral health services show changes on these outcome variables.

TREATMENT

This section describes general models of behavioral health-care service delivery and provides information about specific models of effective EBP delivery approaches.

Models and Processes of Behavioral Health-Care Delivery: Integrated Care

A significant barrier to gaining access to older adults in need of behavioral health services is that older adults rarely utilize outpatient mental health service and community mental health centers (Smyer & Qualls, 1999, p. 15). Older adults are more likely than younger individuals to seek mental health care from their primary care doctor than from a mental health professional (Mickus, Colenda, & Hogan, 2000). Therefore, although disseminating EBPs to these health-care systems is clearly an important agenda, a greater number of older adults will likely be impacted if EBPs are delivered within systems in which older adults present more frequently, namely, primary health care. Much of the current literature that addresses ways to improve older adults' access to behavioral health care suggests that a greater degree of integration between behavioral and primary health care is necessary (Bartels, 2003; HMO Workgroup on Care Management, 2002).

Integration of services can occur in a number of ways. McIntyre (2004) described five different models for integrating behavioral and primary health care. The first model is the *enhanced referral* model. In this model, behavioral health and primary care are physically separated and the primary care physician makes a referral if he or she believes the patient would benefit from behavioral health services. What makes the referral "enhanced" is that the primary care physician makes a referral to a specific behavioral health provider and an attempt is made to get the patient an appointment relatively quickly. However, transportation difficulties and stigma associated with seeing mental health providers has generally resulted in high no-show rates (McIntyre, 2004).

A second model of integration involves behavioral health professionals providing *training to primary care professionals* with the goal of improving detection of common behavioral health concerns of the elderly and increasing referrals. Although this model makes intuitive sense and may make primary health-care workers more sensitive to behavioral health concerns, it has generally proven ineffective in terms of improving detection rates and increasing compliance with clinical practice guidelines (Bartels, 2003).

A third model of integration is *consultation*, a system in which the opinions of behavioral health providers are sought out concerning particular cases that are identified in primary care. This model allows the behavioral health provider more access to patients, but only those cases that are detected in primary care. A major drawback of this model is that detection of behavioral health concerns in primary care may be relatively poor due to the many demands placed on physicians.

Co-location of primary and behavioral health is a fourth option for integration. This model can significantly improve access for patients because the behavioral health-care worker is available on-site within primary care. Patients can be seen on the same day as their primary care appointments, thus reducing the total number of visits. Reducing the number of visits is particularly important for older adults who may have transportation difficulties or physical health concerns that make it difficult to keep numerous appointments. Despite these advantages, behavioral health providers may have difficulties given that they generally lack training in key areas such as rapid assessment and case formulation, disease management, psychopharmacology, treatment adherence, and how to serve as a consultant to primary care physicians (O'Donohue, Cummings, & Ferguson, 2003). Simply placing behavioral health providers in primary care settings without specialized training in how to most effectively provide services in such a setting may not improve service delivery.

Finally, there is the *collaboration* model of integration. In this model, not only is the behavioral health-care worker on-site, but this person is fully integrated into primary care and has specialized training in providing services within a primary care system. This model represents a true team approach to health care and places little emphasis on the distinction between physical illness and mental illness. It shares the primary advantage of the co-location model (i.e., improved access to behavioral health services) and may also reduce stigma since the behavioral health-care provider is on-site and is presented to patients as simply another member of the health-care team. The collaboration model is being increasingly emphasized in the health-care system, particularly in large health maintenance organizations (HMOs). There is evidence that this model may be more effective for delivering EBPs to older adults with behavioral health concerns (Unutzer et al., 2002; Levkoff et al., 2004; Bartels et al., 2004a).

Models and Processes of Behavioral Health-Care Delivery: Other Models

Although integrating primary and behavioral health care has many advantages, there are other models and processes for delivery of EBPs to older adults. For example, community-based outreach programs that target vulnerable older adults in high density areas represent a different model (Katz & Coyne, 2000). This model places an emphasis on taking a more active role in educating individuals in community settings in which older adults typically spend time (e.g., public housing sites, churches, senior centers). Unfortunately, few community-based outreach programs have been subjected to empirical investigation.

Effective EPB Delivery Approaches

We now turn to a discussion of some model programs of EBP service delivery approaches. Many of these model programs represent the collaborative model of service delivery just described because this model has received more empirical examination. Given that other chapters in this book describe specific EBPs in more detail, the following discussion focuses more on the service delivery process and outcomes that have been achieved as opposed to discussing the content of the intervention(s) delivered. The programs described may serve as models for other health-care systems.

Co-Location Models

Although Veterans Affairs (VA) Medical Centers do not provide care exclusively to older adults, a significant proportion of veterans (approximately 37%) are over the age of 65 (Richardson & Waldrop, 2003). The VA Mental

Illness Research, Education, and Clinical Centers (MIRECCs) are designed to meet the unique behavioral health needs of veterans. MIRECCs are behavioral health research and clinical centers located within a larger medical center, making them examples of a co-location model.

As the name implies, MIRECCs conduct research as well as provide direct clinical services. A total of 10 Veterans Integrated Service Networks (VISNs) have MIRECC sites. Each MIRECC site has a specialty ranging from substance dependence, posttraumatic stress disorder, schizophrenia, suicide prevention, and Alzheimer's disease. While each of the individual sites may specialize in a different disorder or combination of disorders, they all focus on the same underlying goal of bringing research findings into practice in order to offer veterans the most effective and up-to-date treatment options. See the National MIRECC Web site (www.mirecc.med.va.gov) for more detailed information about each MIRECC site and the services they offer.

Collaborative Care Models for Depression

There are few well-developed collaborative care programs that are specifically designed to improve the detection and treatment of behavioral health concerns in older adults. Katon and his colleagues (1996) at Group Health Cooperative in Seattle, however, developed a model program for improving the detection and treatment of depression in primary care patients (not exclusively older adults). This intervention involved educating both patients and physicians about EBPs for depression. In addition, patients were involved in a structured depression program delivered in the primary care setting that lasted three to six weeks (2.5 to 3.5 of total direct contact hours). Patients were provided brief evidence-based psychotherapies for depression, had depression scores monitored at each visit, and were monitored for medication side effects. Collaboration with primary care was achieved by providing physicians with consultation notes on the same day that patients received psychotherapy services. Patients receiving these services had lower depression scores and better adherence to antidepressant medications, and rated the quality of their care as good to excellent when compared to a usual care group (Katon et al., 1996).

A study funded by the Hartford Foundation investigated a version of the collaborative model developed by Katon to improve depression management specifically for older adults (Unutzer et al., 2002). In this program, called Improving Mood Promoting Access to Collaborative Treatment (IMPACT), patients are initially screened in primary care clinics and then referred to a depression care manager. Depression care managers in conjunction with the primary care physician then develop an evidence-based treatment plan (i.e., education about depression, initiate medications or problem-solving therapy). The program also involves symptom monitoring and monitoring adherence to the care plan. IMPACT patients reported greater satisfaction with depression care, lower overall depression, better physical and social functioning, and greater quality of life (Unutzer et al., 2002). IMPACT has been recognized as a model program in the report of President's New Freedom Commission on Mental Health (2002).

Bruce and associates (2004) investigated a program similar to IMPACT that targeted not only depressive symptoms, but suicidal ideation. Their program, called Prevention of Suicide in Primary Care Elderly Collaborative Trial (PROSPECT), involves two main components: educating primary care physicians by providing a clinical algorithm for treating geriatric depression and providing evidence-based treatment. Treatment was provided by depression care managers and included selective serotonin reuptake inhibitor medications or interpersonal psychotherapy. Depression care managers assisted physicians in diagnosing depression, offered treatment recommendations, monitored clinical status, and provided follow-up care. Results indicated that PROSPECT patients showed greater and more rapid declines in suicidal ideation and greater and more rapid reductions in depression (Bruce et al., 2004).

Other large HMOs have implemented similar programs for managing depression in their older members. For example, Sierra Health Services screens patients using the 15-item GDS. Positive screens for either major or minor depression are referred to a behavioral health program, situational counseling, or a support group. Studies indicate that 70% of patients no longer meet criteria for depression following treatment (HMO Workgroup on Care Management, 2002).

Collaborative Care Models for Severe Mental Illness

Bartels and colleagues (2004b) developed an integrated care model of EBP delivery for older adults suffering from severe mental illness (SMI). Their model is somewhat different from those programs for depression, however. Older adults with SMI often have undetected comorbid medical problems and have difficulties engaging in effective self-care practices, which places them at higher risk for institutionalization (Bartels, Muesser, & Miles, 1997; Bartels et al., 2004b). Therefore, their model is more concerned with integrating primary health care into behavioral health care instead of the other way around.

Services provided in this model involve two major components: skills training and health maintenance. The skills training program is based on

EBPs for younger individuals with SMI and is provided in a group format. Skills training groups focus on teaching life skills such as effective communication with health-care providers, handling medications, illness self-management, and basic social skills. The health maintenance program is designed to assesses chronic health-care needs, track and promote the use of preventive primary care, facilitate health-care visits, document medical needs and services provided, and detect untreated health-care concerns (e.g., need for eyeglasses). Both sets of services are provided by a nurse case manager.

In a small outcome study investigating the effectiveness of this model, Bartels and colleagues (2004b) found that individuals receiving both skills training and health maintenance (ST+HM) showed improved social functioning and independent living skills compared to a group that received only an HM intervention. In addition, patients in the ST+MH and the HM conditions demonstrated an increased use of preventive health services and identification of previously undetected medical disorders (Bartels et al., 2004b). A larger study is underway that will examine this service delivery model in greater detail (e.g., whether this model delays institutionalization) and with a much larger sample.

Collaborative Care Models for Dementia

Families of older adults with dementia often need a variety of services to most effectively manage the numerous stresses associated with caregiving, planning for the future, and providing care for the patient at home. Services include not only appropriate medical care for the dementia patient, but additional services such as education, case management, respite care, legal services, and support groups. Because one health-care system often cannot provide all of these services, several large managed care organizations in California have developed partnerships with local community agencies to increase the likelihood that families will take advantage of available services (HMO Workgroup on Care Management, 2002). Important agencies include local chapters of the Alzheimer's Association and Caregiver Resource Centers (there are a total of 11 centers in California) that provide evidence-based counseling and education programs for family caregivers. Families are able to complete one Web-based intake form that includes relevant information for all community agencies. Families then are able to provide permission for this information to be shared among the agencies so that appropriate services can be offered. A similar program is available in Colorado through Centura Life Center (HMO Workgroup on Care Management, 2002).

These programs represent well-coordinated efforts between primary care and a variety of community-based agencies. Evidence-based services for family caregivers may be provided through local chapters of the Alzheimer's Association, the National Family Caregiver Support Program (guided by state Administrations on Aging), or other state-based service programs (e.g., the Nevada Caregiver Support Center, the Older Adult and Family Center in Palo Alto, CA). These efforts to coordinate primary care and community-based social services can reduce burden on families and assist families with navigating complex social service systems. Furthermore, comprehensive family support and counseling can delay institutionalization (Mittelman et al., 1993).

Other Collaborative Care Models

Programs of All-Inclusive Care for the Elderly (PACE) utilize multidisciplinary teams involving primary care physicians, nurses, dieticians, drivers, social workers, and rehabilitation staff to provide cost-effective and comprehensive health-care services to the elderly (Lee, Eng, Fox, & Etienne, 1998). The philosophy of the program involves improving overall quality of life while also helping individuals remain in their homes and communities for as long as possible. The expense of hospitals and nursing home stays is unaffordable for many, and cost the government a substantial amount of money.

PACE remains financially viable by pooling federal assistance funds (e.g., Medicare and Medicaid) to provide the appropriate care for patients. Pooling the funds in this manner allows the money to be used for health-care services that may not have been covered if funds had been collected by the individual services (e.g., social services interventions, transportation to appointments, adult day care, respite care, extended home nursing care) rather than by the comprehensive care program. Additionally, this monetary discretion allows PACE to provide more flexible, individual, and patient-focused care (Lee et al., 1998).

Individuals eligible for PACE must be at least 55 years of age, need assistance in carrying out several activities of daily living (e.g., bathing, cooking, managing money), have numerous medical conditions, and be eligible to receive Medicare and Medicaid (Lee et al., 1998). Although these individuals are usually still living in the community, they are considered high risk and vulnerable because they are likely to require either hospitalizations or nursing home care (Lee et al., 1998). There is also a significant percentage (42%) of those utilizing PACE who have a diagnosis of some type of dementia (Miller, Miller, Mauser, & O'Malley, 1997).

Enrolled individuals have access to any services that are deemed necessary following a comprehensive assessment. Care provided in PACE is outcome oriented; the team sets goals for each individual, which are assigned to the member of the team who can most directly make progress toward the fulfillment of the goal (Miller et al., 1997). Sometimes mental health services are determined to be necessary. In fact, one of the most common adjustments made in initial care plans is the identification of mental health issues such as depression, anxiety, and dementia (Miller et al., 1997). Thus, although mental health professionals are not an immediate part of the PACE team, mental health services are provided on a case-by-case basis.

To date, there have been several outcome studies evaluating the effectiveness of PACE. Miller et al. (1997) found that while individuals enrolled in the program were more likely to use ambulatory-care visits, hospitals and nursing homes were used less often. These authors also found that PACE seemed to be better suited for those with more functional limitations while those with dementia were more likely to discontinue use of the program. Chatterji, Burstein, Kidder, and White (1998) completed an exhaustive evaluation of PACE examining several outcomes including the use of support services (e.g., attending day health center), use of medical services (e.g., nursing home visits or inpatient hospital stays), patient satisfaction, health status, mortality, and quality of life. Similar to the findings of Miller and associates (1997), individuals with the most severe conditions seem to benefit the most from the program.

These collaborative care approaches to delivering EBPs are promising and should serve as models for others, as they provide primary care with needed support and behavioral health expertise. These interventions have been implemented not only in large HMOs, but also in general primary care settings. Similar programs could be developed for delivering EBPs for other conditions such as anxiety disorders or substance abuse.

State-Based Programs for Dual Diagnosis

In 2002, the Substance Abuse and Mental Health Service Administration (SAMHSA) reported to Congress information about state-based innovative prevention and intervention services (e.g., integrated treatment) for individuals with co-occurring substance abuse and mental health concerns. Two states described programs that targeted older adults (Wisconsin and California). The Wisconsin program was designed to serve older adults with dual diagnoses. Regional training sessions were completed that emphasized improving coordination of mental health and substance abuse services as well enhancing integrated treatment. California also targeted individuals (not just elders) with dual diagnoses. Coordination of substance abuse and mental health services improved psychiatric functioning, access to mental health treatment, quality of life, physical health treatment, and decreased substance abuse.

Studies Comparing Service Delivery Models

There is only one study that compared the effectiveness of the different models of integration previously described. Hedrick and colleagues (2003) compared a collaborative care (CC) model of service delivery with a consult-liaison (CL) care model within a VA primary care clinic. In the CL condition, primary care providers were responsible for identifying cases of depression and consulting with or referring to a mental health provider, as necessary. The CC model involved a team of mental health providers meeting weekly to develop treatment and evaluation plans for patients. Frequent contact with primary care providers was achieved via electronic notes and personal contacts. In the CC model, evidence-based interventions (e.g., medication, cognitive behavior therapy) were implemented in a stepwise fashion, with the least resource-intensive interventions provided first. Overall, the CC model involved a greater degree of contact between primary care and behavioral health providers, the involvement of a team of behavioral health-care providers, explicit implementation of EBPs in a stepwise manner, and more frequent evaluation of patient progress. Results indicated that the CC model led to more rapid improvement in depressive symptoms and an increased proportion of patients receiving EBPs. This study provides some initial data supporting the superiority of the CC model of service delivery for older adults with depression.

An ongoing study called the Primary Care Research in Substance Abuse and Mental Health Services for the Elderly (PRISM-E) is comparing an integrated care model with a service model involving referral to mental health or substance abuse providers outside of the primary care setting (McIntyre, 2004). The PRISM-E study represents the largest study to date of depression and alcohol abuse in older adults and is the first to compare integration and referral models of service delivery. Outcomes being examined include clinical as well as cost outcomes. The PRISM-E study has yet to be completed, but is now in its sixth and final year; data will be forthcoming.

PREVENTION AND OUTREACH

The health-care system lacks programs designed to prevent mental illness in older adults (Bartels, 2003). Some outreach programs, however, have been developed that involve delivering EBPs with the goal of preventing high rates of primary health-care utilization as well as preventing emotional suffering. Cummings (1997) described two early outreach programs that were delivered within the context of a behavioral health-care delivery system (i.e., American Biodyne) that was integrated with Medicare providers. The first was a bereavement program that involved contacting patients within two weeks of losing their loved one. A series of 14, two-hour therapy groups specially designed to address bereavement issues were provided to those in the experimental group, and all patients were followed for two years. Results indicated that the bereavement program resulted in a savings of $1,400 per patient over the two-year period and resulted in reduced physical and emotional suffering (Cummings, 1997).

In the second program, Cummings (1997) instituted an early Alzheimer's counseling program. The program was designed to meet the needs of both caregivers and Alzheimer's patients. Services included teaching relaxation and guided imagery skills, education about the disease, and continuous access to a hotline for advice and emotional support. Caregivers were also instructed to carry the names of three individuals whom they could call if they felt overwhelmed. Those in the intervention group demonstrated reductions in emergency room visits, inpatient hospital days, and nighttime phone calls in the year following involvement in this program compared to the year prior to starting the program. These programs serve as models for future outreach programs within primary care systems. They also demonstrate the impact that evidence-based psychosocial interventions can have on improving both emotional functioning and reducing costs associated with high health-care utilization.

Few empirically supported community-based outreach models for delivering EBPs to older adults with behavioral health concerns exist. Rabins and colleagues (2000), however, developed and investigated a community-based program called the Psychogeriatric Assessment and Treatment in City Housing (PATCH) program. This program, targeting older adults living in public housing developments, included three components: educating building staff (e.g., managers, social workers, groundskeepers) to be case finders; performing behavioral health screenings and assessments; and providing evidence-based care when indicated (e.g., education about medication management, counseling, education concerning health management). Assessment and treatment services were provided in the individual's home by a nurse. Results indicated that the PATCH intervention was more effective in reducing psychiatric symptoms than a usual care control group.

Raschko (1990) described a model similar to the PATCH program. This gatekeeper model involved training individuals in the community who frequently interact with potentially at-risk elderly individuals (e.g., postal workers, telephone company personnel, and bank personnel). Once at-risk individuals were identified and referred to health-care providers, elders received multidisciplinary in-home assessment, intervention, and case management. Interventions included medical, psychiatric, and socioeconomic components. Few outcomes were reported, but the program increased recognition of high-risk elders.

DISCUSSION AND CONCLUSIONS

The primary goal of this chapter is to describe the most effective ways in which EBPs for older adults suffering from behavioral health concerns are currently delivered. At this point in time, there are still few empirically supported approaches for delivering EBPs to older adults with behavioral health concerns. It appears as if models designed to fully integrate behavioral and primary care can have positive effects on a variety of outcomes. In addition, models for identifying and treating elderly individuals in the community are a viable means for serving those individuals who are not likely to utilize primary health care. Unfortunately, little research has been conducted investigating these community-based approaches.

The delivery of EBPs clearly requires more than simply providing education and referral information to older adults, physicians, or other community members. Behavioral health-care workers need to position themselves in places in which older adults are likely to present and where they prefer being treated (i.e., in primary care or in the community). Furthermore, successful service delivery should include the following components: more aggressive follow-up with attention to treatment adherence, early recognition of adverse effects of medication, and modification of interventions as needed (Katz & Coyne, 2000). One innovative method by which to enhance service delivery is the toolkit. SAMHSA has developed a series of these toolkits for six different EBPs (i.e., illness management and recovery; medication management approaches in psychiatry; assertive community treatment; family psychoeducation; supported employment; and integrated duel diagnosis treatment). Toolkits are designed for practitioners, clients, families, program leaders, and administrators. They include a wide range of educational materials such as information sheets for different stakeholders, introductory and practice demonstration videos, and manuals and implementation tips for practitioners, as well as outcome measures and fidelity scales to facilitate implementation of EBPs. As has been discussed throughout this book, changing the practices of health-care providers is one of the most difficult challenges to improving recognition and treatment of behavioral health concerns in older adults. Implementation of these comprehensive and detailed toolkits is one more method for creating change in the practice of clinicians (Bartels et al., 2002). More information about these toolkits can be obtained from the SAMHSA Web site (www.samhsa.gov).

It is clear that further research designed to improve EBP delivery is needed. Fortunately, some exciting work is underway. Results from the PRISM-E project described herein will be available in the near future, providing much-needed data on integrated service delivery compared to a more traditional referral-based model. Also, in 2002 the Center for Mental Health Services awarded nine grants as part of their Targeted Capacity Expansion (TCE) grant program. TCE grants are designed, in part, to improve implementation of evidence-based mental health practices to older adults. Evaluations of each of the nine programs will be conducted and results may prove useful to other communities who wish to design similar programs. Finally, the National Council on the Aging's Positive Aging Act was introduced in June of 2004 that, if approved, would provide funding to states and nonprofit organizations to integrate behavioral health screening and treatment into primary care settings. All of these efforts should increase our understanding of how to best deliver EBPs to an ever-growing number of older adults who suffer from mental health conditions.

REFERENCES

Bartels, S. J. (2003). Improving the system of care for older adults with mental illness in the United States: Findings and recommendations for the president's new Freedom Commission on mental health. *American Journal of Geriatric Psychiatry, 11*, 486–497.

Bartels, S. J., Dums, A. R., Oxman, T. E., Schneider, L. S., Areán, P. A., Alexopoulos, G. S., & Jeste, D. V. (2002). Evidence-based practices in geriatric mental health care. *Psychiatric Services, 53*, 1419–1431.

Bartels, S. J., Coakley, E. H., Zubritsky, C., Ware, J. H., Miles, K. M., Areán, P. A., et al. (2004a). Improving access to geriatric mental health services: A randomized trial comparing treatment engagement in integrated and enhanced referral care for depression, anxiety, and at-risk alcohol use. *American Journal of Psychiatry, 161*, 1455–1462.

Bartels, S. J., Forester, B., Mueser, K. T., Miles, K. M., Dums, A. R., Pratt, S. I. et al. (2004b). Enhanced skills training and health care management for older persons with severe mental illness. *Community Mental Health Journal, 40*, 75–90.

Bartels, S. J., Muesser, K. T., & Miles, K. M. (1997). A comparative study of elderly patients with schizophrenia and bipolar disorder in nursing homes and the community. *Schizophrenia Research, 27*, 181–190.

Beck, A. T., Ward, C. H., Mendelson, M., Mock, J., & Erbaugh, J. (1961). An inventory for measuring depression. *Archives of General Psychiatry, 4*, 561–571.

Bruce, M. L., Ten Have, T. R., Reynolds, C. F., Katz, I. I., Schulberg, H. C., Mulsant, B. H., et al. (2004). Reducing suicidal ideation and depressive symptoms in depressed older primary care patients. *Journal of the American Medical Association, 291*, 1081–1091.

Butcher, J. N., Dahlstrom, W. G., Graham, J. R., Tellgen, A., & Kaemmer, B. (1989). *Minnesota Multiphasic Personality Inventory-2 (MMPI-2): Manual for administration and scoring.* Minneapolis, MN: University of Minnesota Press.

Chambless, D. L., Baker, M. J., Baucom, D. H., Beutler, L. E., Calhoun, K. S., Crits-Christoph, P., et al. (1998). Update on empirically-validated therapies II. *Clinical Psychologist, 51*, 3–16.

Chatterji, P., Burstein, N. R., Kidder, D., & White, A. J. (1998). *Evaluation of the program of all-inclusive care for the elderly (PACE) demonstration: The impact of PACE on particular outcome (FINAL).* Washington, D.C.: Health Care Financing Administration.

Cummings, N. A. (1997). Approaches to preventive care. In P. E. Hartman-Stein (Ed.), *Innovative behavioral healthcare for older adults: A guidebook for changing times* (pp. 1–17). San Francisco: Jossey-Bass.

Ewing, J. A. (1984). Detecting alcoholism: The CAGE questionnaire. *Journal of the American Medical Association, 252*, 1905–1907.

First, M. B., Spitzer, R. L., Gibbon, M., & Williams, J. B. W. (1996). *User's guide for the structured clinical interview for DSM-IV Axis I Disorders (SCID-I) Research Version.* New York: Biometrics Research.

Gatz, M., Fiske, A., Fox, L. S., Kaskie, B., Kasl-Godley, J. E., McCallum, T. J., & Wetherell, J. L. (1998). Empirically validated psychological treatments for older adults. *Journal of Mental Health and Aging, 4*, 9–46.

Hayes, S. C., Barlow, D. H., & Nelson-Gray, R. O. (1999). *The scientist practitioner: Research and accountability in the age of managed care.* Boston: Allyn and Bacon.

Hedrick, S. C., Chaney, E. F., Felker, B., Liu, C., Hasenberg, N., Heaggerty, P., et al. (2003). Effectiveness of collaborative care depression treatment in veterans' affairs primary care. *Journal of General Internal Medicine, 18*, 9–16.

HMO Workgroup on Care Management. (2002). *Improving the care of older adults with common geriatric conditions.* Washington, DC: AAHP Foundation.

Katon, W., Robinson, P., Von Korff, M., Lin, E., Bush, T., Ludman, E., et al. (1996). A multifaceted intervention to improve treatment of depression in primary care. *Archives of General Psychiatry, 53*, 924–932.

Katz, I. I., & Coyne, J. C. (2000). The public health model for mental health care for the elderly. *Journal of the American Medical Association, 283*, 2844–2845.

Lee, W., Eng, C., Fox, N., & Etienne, M. (1998). PACE: A model for integrated care of frail older patients. *Geriatrics, 53*, 62–67.

Levkoff, S. E., Chen, H., Coakley, E., McDonel Herr, E. C., Oslin, D. W., Katz, I., et al. (2004). Design and sample characteristics of the PRISM-E multisite randomized trial to improve behavioral health care for the elderly. *Journal of Aging and Health, 16*(1), 3–27.

Lichtenberg, P. A. (1999). *Handbook of assessment in clinical gerontology.* New York: Wiley.

McIntyre, J. (2004). *Integrating mental health into primary care.* Web seminar presented on March 9, 2004, at http://www.asaging.org/webseminars/websem.cfm? EventID=8125.

Mickus, M., Colenda, C. C., & Hogan, A. J. (2000). Knowledge of mental health benefits and preferences for type of mental health providers among the general public. *Psychiatric Services, 51,* 199–202.

Miller, S. N., Miller, N. A., Mauser, E., & O'Malley, K. (1997). PACE: Innovative care for the frail older adult. In P. E. Hartman-Stein (Ed.), *Innovative behavioral healthcare for older adults: A guidebook for changing times* (pp. 19–39). San Francisco: Jossey-Bass.

Mittelman, M. S., Ferris, S. H. Steinberg, G., Shulman, E., Mackell, J. A., Ambiner, A., et al. (1993). An intervention that delays institutionalization of Alzheimer's disease patients: Treatment of spouse-caregivers. *Gerontologist, 33,* 730–740.

O'Donohue, W. T., Buchanan, J. A., & Fisher, J. E. (2000). Characteristics of empirically-supported treatments. *Journal of Psychotherapy Research and Practice, 9,* 69–74.

O'Donohue, W. T., Cummings, N. A., & Ferguson, K. F. (2003). Clinical integration: The promise and the path. In N. A. Cummings, W. T. O'Donohue and K. F. Ferguson (Eds.), *Behavioral health as primary care: Beyond efficacy to effectiveness* (pp. 15–30). Reno, NV: Context Press.

President's New Freedom Commission on Mental Health. (2002). In Executive Order 13263.

Rabins, P. V., Black, B. S., Roca, R., German, P., McGuire, M., Robbins, B., et al. (2000). Effectiveness of a nurse-based outreach program for identifying and treating psychiatric illness in the elderly. *Journal of the American Medical Association, 283,* 2802–2809.

Raschko, R. (1990). The gatekeeper model for the isolated at-risk elderly. In N. L. Cohen (Ed.), *Psychiatry takes to the streets* (pp. 195–209). New York: Guilford.

Richardson, C., & Waldrop, J. (2003). *Veterans: 2000 Census 2000 brief.* Retrieved February 11, 2004, from http://www.va.gov/vetdata/Census2000/c2kbr-22.pdf.

Smyer, M. A., & Qualls, S. H. (1999). *Aging and mental health.* Malden, MA: Blackwell.

Stanley, M. A., & Beck, J. G. (2000). Anxiety disorders. *Clinical Psychology Review, 20,* 731–754.

Unutzer, J., Katon, W., Callahan, C. M., Williams, J. W., Hunkeler, E., Harpole, L., et al. (2002). Collaborative care management of late-life depression in the primary care setting. *Journal of the American Medical Association, 288,* 2836–2845.

U.S. Department of Health and Human Services. (1999). *Mental health: A report of the Surgeon General.* Rockville, MD: Author.

Whooley, M. A., Avins, A. L., Miranda, J., & Browner, W. S. (1997). Case-finding instruments for depression: Two questions are as good as many. *Journal of General Internal Medicine, 12,* 439–445.

Yesavage, J. A., Brink, T. L., Rose, T. L., Lum, O., Huang, V., Adey, M., et al. (1983). Development and validation of a geriatric depression screening scale: A preliminary report. *Journal of Psychiatric Research, 17,* 37–49.

CHAPTER 8

Evidence-Based Practices Within Special Settings

John M. Worrall, Stacey Cherup, Ruth A. Gentry, Jane E. Fisher, and Hillary LeRoux

FAITH-BASED ORGANIZATIONS

Since the days of Florence Nightingale, religious institutions have been involved in medicine and health promotion. Florence Nightingale emphasized the need for nursing to honor the psychological and spiritual aspects of patients in promoting health (Nightingale, 1860 in Peterson, Atwood, & Yates, 2002), and the tradition continues today with faith-based organizations running many of the nation's hospitals.

Religion is an integral part of the lives of the majority of the elderly in the United States. Nearly two-thirds of them report that religion is very important in their lives; half attend religious services once a week or more (Benjamins, 2004). Religious beliefs and practices consistently have been shown to have a positive effect on behavioral health and well-being (Coyle, 2001; Harrison, Koenig & Hays, 2001). Engaging in private religious activities, such as prayer, meditation, or Bible study, has been shown to improve longevity. In a 6-year study of 3,851 older adults who participated in private religious activity prior to the onset of activities of daily living (ADL) impairment, participants had a survival advantage over those who did not (Helm, Hays, & Flint, 2000). Frequent participation in religious services is also associated with positive health outcomes. A 29-year long longitudinal study of 2,676 individuals found weekly religious attendance to be associated with improving or maintaining good mental health, supportive social relationships, and marital stability (Strawbridge, Shema, & Cohen, 2001). In another study, McCullough, Hoyt, and Larson (2000) found a positive correlation between religious involvement and lifespan. Benjamins (2004) found that religious attendance predicted fewer functional limitations.

Faith-Based Behavioral Health Interventions

Interventions that incorporate religious and spiritual ideas and teachings into the therapeutic process have proliferated in recent years. They are not necessarily designed solely for people professing particular religious or spiritual beliefs. For instance, Alcoholics Anonymous (AA) and other twelve-step programs have their roots in spiritual beliefs and practices.

This section reviews faith-based services and practices that influence behavioral health outcomes. The faith-based behavioral health programs may or may not incorporate religious and spiritual ideas and teachings into their service. For the purposes of this review, "empirically supported" means that efficacy has been demonstrated in a controlled setting, for example, with a randomized clinical trial, and that clinical effectiveness and cost-effectiveness have been demonstrated in the field (Chambless & Hollon, 1998).

Church-Based Health Promotion Programs

Peterson, Atwood, and Yates (2002) reviewed church-based health promotion programs (CBHPPs) in order to identify variables that accounted for the effectiveness of CBHPP's positive outcomes in promoting emotional, physical, and spiritual health. They identified seven key elements:

1. Churches effectively established partnerships with health-care organizations, particularly in underserved communities.
2. Clergy were able to influence congregations to undertake positive lifestyle changes.
3. Churches are in virtually every community in the United States, with 60% of individuals having some involvement with a church.
4. Churches have a strong base of volunteers willing to train as health-promotion leaders.
5. Many churches serve strong social, educational, and political functions in the community.
6. Churches promote healthy behavior change while incorporating traditional cultural values.
7. Churches typically provide supportive social relationships to facilitate behavior change.

Faith-Based Self-Help Programs

Americans make more visits to self-help groups for substance abuse and psychiatric problems than to all mental health professionals combined. Seven percent of Americans reported attending a self-help group for some problem in the previous twelve months (Kessler, Mickelson, & Zhao, 1997 in Humphreys, Wing, & McCarty, 2004).

Research on outcomes of Alcoholics Anonymous and Narcotics Anonymous participants found that these self-help groups are effective in reducing substance abuse and lowering health-care costs. These groups are also effective at enhancing individual self-efficacy, improving social support, reducing depression and anxiety, and helping individuals to cope more effectively with stress (Humphreys, Wing, & McCarty, 2004).

PRIMARY CARE

Since the mid-1970s, epidemiologic research on mental disorders indicates that primary care is the first setting in the mental health-care delivery system in which individuals present with mental health problems (Simon & Vonkorff, 1997; Mauer, 2003; Peek & Heinrich, 2000). The National Institutes of Mental Health Epidemiologic Catchment Area Study found that about 50% of care for common mental disorders is delivered in general medical settings (Mauer, 2003). Surveys have found that 70% of primary care visits were psychosocial in nature (Fries, Koop, & Beadle, 1993; Strosahl, 2002). An older person who is in psychological distress is more likely to visit his or her primary care physician than any other provider (Speer & Schneider, 2003); however the physician may lack the time, training, or experience to adequately detect or treat the older person's mental health problem (Kaplan, Adamek, & Martin, 2001).

In spite of a significant amount of contact between older adults and primary care professionals, many behavioral health problems are undiagnosed and undertreated in primary care settings (Mauer, 2003; Simon & Vonkorff, 1997). For example, a large percentage of elderly persons who commit suicide have had recent contact with their primary care physician: 20% of seniors had been seen by a physician within 24 hours of committing suicide; 35% within one week of committing suicide; 75% within one month of committing suicide; and 80% within six months of committing suicide (American Association of Suicidology, 2002). Ninety percent of older adults exhibiting suicidal behavior have diagnosable depression (Conwell, 1997 in Kaplan, Adamek, & Martin, 2001). Timely diagnosis and an appropriate referral is likely to reduce suffering and save money on future health-care utilization costs, and may ultimately prevent a suicide.

Research indicates that the currently used screening methods, treatment guidelines and procedures, and provider education programs on mental health have been ineffective in helping primary care health-care workers identify mental health problems (Mauer, 2003). Research focused on the application of evidence-based practices (EBPs) in both primary care settings and specialty mental health settings indicates that the use of specific assessment in treatment techniques will result in better outcomes for patients (Mauer, 2003). *Integrated care* is one model in which the use of EBPs has been successfully implemented and improved patient care in primary care settings.

Integrated Care

What Is Integrated Care?

Integrated care involves collaboration of mental health professionals within a primary care setting to create a coordinated, multidisciplinary team in which mental health professionals (e.g., psychologists and social workers) and medical professionals, such as pediatricians, internists, and nurse practitioners, work together (Aitken & Curtis, 2004; Cucciare, in press). More specifically, integrated care is "a service that combines medical and behavioral [e.g., mental] health services to more fully address the spectrum of problems that patients bring to their primary medical care providers" (Blount, 1998, p. 1). It is a set of techniques and organizational models designed to produce connectivity, alignment, and collaboration both within and across providers (e.g., both health-care and mental health-care workers) and insurance companies (e.g., the funding and administrative levels) to provide necessary and appropriate care for patients (Kodner, 2000).

The delivery of integrated care is most effective when behavioral health services are provided in the primary care setting (e.g., mental health professionals work in the same office as the health-care provider) (Aitken & Curtis, 2004). Many health-care systems have been experimenting with integrated care providing support for the use of this model in improving patient care (Kirchner, Cody, Thrush, Sullivan, & Rapp, 2004).

Table 8.1 provides a comparison of integrated health care and the current health-care system in which the health-care worker will refer the patient to a specialty mental health service (Baker & Braddie, 1997; Strosahl et al., 1997; O'Donohue et al., 2006).

The goals of integrated care are to:

- Increase the quality of patient care.
- Enhance the patient's qualify of life.
- Improve consumer satisfaction.
- Build a health-care system that is efficient and effective for patients with multiple, complex problems present across multiple sectors and

TABLE 8.1   Integrated Care versus Specialty Mental Health Care

Dimension/Feature	Integrated Behavioral Health Care	Specialty Mental Health Care (current health-care system)
Mission	Primary care service focused on behavioral/mental health issues	Specialty mental health care provided separately from primary care (e.g., referrals)
Delivery location	Part of primary care services; found in the medical practice area	Specialized service offered in a separate location
Who provides care	Health-care provider	Therapist or mental health worker
Type of care provided	Consultation session approximately 15–30 minutes long and usually one to three sessions of care	Psychotherapy sessions usually 50 minutes long; length of treatment varies by problem(s)
Structure of care	Behavioral health provider is part of primary care team	Therapist is separate from the primary care setting; works alone or as part of the specialty mental health team
Primary customers	Health-care worker, then patient, in press	Patient, then all others

providers (e.g., a patient with cancer and an anxiety disorder can easily obtain needed care) (Kodner, 2000).

- Reduce health-care costs by maintaining patient good health and preventing a health crisis by implementing early and appropriate interventions for illnesses and illness-producing behaviors (Slay & McLeod, 1997).

Why Use Integrated Care?

Problems with Current Health-Care System. Both the health-care systems (e.g., primary care physicians, specialists, nurses, and hospitals) and social-care systems (e.g., social services, home based care, and specialty mental health—outpatient and inpatient) in the United States are fragmented and uncoordinated (Kodner, 2000). Many jurisdictions, agencies, and professionals are responsible for providing care, making the ability of both patients and health-care providers to deliver and obtain effective and efficient care difficult and complex (Kodner, 2000). Without an integrated care system, overlap between services results and important patient needs are left unmet (e.g., unnecessary hospitalization may occur, institutionalization rates rise, quality of care diminishes, and costs are poorly controlled; Kodner, 2000). Additionally, research indicates that many patients with mental health problems are unrecognized and untreated in medical settings due to the current organization of the health-care system (Simon & Vonkorff, 1997). Because of the lack of coordination between services, the economic costs of health care, especially chronic care (e.g., diabetes or arthritis), is enormous (e.g., unrecognized and untreated mental health problems have a major negative impact on daily functioning, work capability, and social functioning) (Kodner, 2000; Simon & Vonkorff, 1997).

Advantages of Integrated Care. Integrated health care avoids many problems found in the current health-care system by providing patients with non-stigmatizing cost-effective care that results in healthier and more satisfied consumers (see O'Donohue et al., 2006). Research indicates that patients often present mental health problems (e.g., depression and anxiety) in a medical setting rather than in a mental health-care setting because there is less stigma associated with being treated by a health-care worker; the medical setting is more convenient and accessible; and health-care workers are generally more trusted (Mauer, 2003; Simon & Vonkorff, 1997). Patients prefer the one-stop shopping model of integrated care, in which treatment for all health-related problems (involving behavioral, lifestyle, and physical features) is available (O'Donohue et al., 2006). Physical and behavioral health problems are often inextricably related. Physical problems can cause or contribute to behavioral health problems and vice versa (e.g., diabetes can result in depression and medications can cause problems like sexual dysfunction; a sedentary lifestyle and poor diet self-control can lead to or exacerbate diabetes. The most commonly prescribed medical treatment for behavioral health problems, psychotropic medications, do not always help patients (Simon & Vonkorff, 1997; Sink, Holden, & Yaffe, 2005). Integrated health care allows patients to choose from an array of treatment options (e.g., psychotropic medications, psychotherapy and/or participation in behavioral health education classes can be offered to a patient presenting with depression). Integrated health care can be more cost-effective by providing patients the care they need instead of the care professionals typically have readily available (O'Donohue et al., 2006; Simon & Vonkorff, 1997). Additionally, integrated health care has been demonstrated to improve detection of a fuller range of patients' problems (e.g., both physical and behavioral), and hence leads to better patient outcomes (O'Donohue et al., 2006). Finally, many physicians report that they are more satisfied with integrated health care (Gallo et al., 2004).

Case Examples of Integrated Care

Several health-care systems have been experimenting with the effectiveness of integrated health care. Examples of studies of effective integrated health-care systems include (1) Kaiser Permanente health system; (2) Group Health Cooperative of Puget Sound; (3) Healthcare Partners in Los Angeles County; (4) United States Air Force; and (5) Veterans Affairs (VA) community-based outpatient clinics (Cummings, 1997; Druss, Rohrbaugh, Levinson, & Rosenheck, 2001; Kirchner et al., 2004; *Primary Behavioral Healthcare Services Practice Manual 2.0.*, 2002; Slay & McLeod, 1997; Simon & Vonkorff, 1997; Strosahl, Baker, Braddick, & Braddick, 1997). In addition, researchers have begun to examine how to implement integrated care systems within rural settings (e.g., VA community-based outpatient clinics) (Kirchner et. al., 2004).

Recently, studies have examined the effectiveness of integrated health care in an older adult population. Examples include collaborative care of depression management in primary care and PRISM-E for depression, anxiety, and at-risk alcohol use (Bartels et al., 2004; Gallo et al., 2004; Unützer et al., 2002).

Overall, the current research supports the use of integrated health care, but the model is not without its problems. For additional information, see the Further Reading and Related Websites section at the end of this chapter.

Barriers to Implementation of the Integrated Model

Several barriers to implementing an integrated health-care model have been described in the literature including:

- The dominant view in medicine and psychology that the "mind" and body are separate and should be treated as separate, this model has been shown to be ineffective in that it results in unrecognized and untreated behavioral and psychological problems (Cummings, 1997).
- The current health-care system predominately uses the carve-out system that involves a fee for service and referrals out to mental health services. Cummings (1997) argues that as long as this system is in place, an integrated care or carve-in system will not be used.
- There is a need for both medical and behavioral (e.g., mental) health-care workers to develop skills to implement interdisciplinary teams needed to implement integrated care effectively (Kirchner et al., 2004).
- Primary care settings do not allow the time necessary to implement integrated care, nor do they have the physical space (Cummings, 1997; Kirchner et al., 2004).

- Lack of emphasis on teamwork and building relationships between medical and behavioral (e.g., mental) health care results in a lack of knowledge about and poor attitudes toward the importance of mental health problems (Kirchner et al., 2004).

Recommendations for Developing Integrated Care Services

Given the barriers to using integrated care, how can integrated care be effectively implemented into a primary care setting? Below are guidelines for implementing integrated care. For more detailed information, see the Further Reading section at the end of this chapter.

Steps to Implementation

- *Staff training.* O'Donohue et al. (2006) caution that integrated care does not involve simply having a mental health work function in a medical setting. They suggest that as a system moves toward an integrated care model, both the medical and behavioral health-care workers will benefit from guidance in performing their respective duties and coordinating care. Behavioral care provider (BCP) training should focus on increasing medical knowledge/literacy and consultation/liaison skills; fostering an understanding of population management, increasing skill needed to perform in a medical culture (i.e., faster, more action-oriented, treatment driven, team-based delivery); increasing knowledge of psychopharmacology; increasing knowledge of medically related assessments and interventions such as disease management and treatment adherence.

How does an integrated care model function? Strosahl (1998) and O'Donohue et al. (2006) provide detailed operational principles for implementing an integrated care model. The operation of an integrated care model involves the seamless coordination of patient care through the collaboration of the treatment team. According to Strosahl, et al. (1997) and O'Donohue et al. (2006) the BCP's role on the team typically requires care competencies for the following services:

- Triage/liaison services: A screening designed to determine the appropriate level of behavioral care for a patient (e.g., primary care versus specialty care versus inpatient care) typically provided that same day during the patient's first visit.
- Consultation: An initial visit by a patient who is referred to the BCP for a general evaluation focusing on diagnostic and functional evaluation,

recommendations for treatment, education for the patient and/or family members, and forming limited behavior change goals.

- Behavioral health follow-up: Secondary visits by a patient to support a behavior change plan or treatment started in a prior consultation visit. These visits often occur in tandem with planned primary care provider (PCP) visits.
- Compliance enhancement: A BCP visit designed to help the patient adhere to an intervention initiated by the PCP. The focus of the visit is on education, addressing negative beliefs, or strategies for coping with medication side effects.
- Relapse prevention: A BCP visit designed to maintain stable functioning in a patient who has responded to previous treatment: Visits are often spaced at longer intervals.
- Behavioral medicine: A BCP may visit to assist patients in managing a chronic medical condition or tolerating an invasive or uncomfortable medical procedure. The focus may be on lifestyle issues or health risk factors among patients at risk (e.g., smoking cessation, stress management, or weight loss) or may involve managing issues related to progressive illness such as end-stage chronic obstructive pulmonary disease (COPD).
- Specialty consultation: A BCP provides consultative services over time to patients whose situations require ongoing monitoring and follow-up. These visits are most applicable to patients with chronic stressors or marginal healthy lifestyle skills.
- Psychoeducational class: The BCP provides brief group treatment that either replaces or supplements individual consultative treatment, and that is designed to promote education and skill building. A psychoeducational group can serve as the primary psychological intervention because many behavioral health needs are best addressed in this type of group treatment.
- Conjoint consultation: The BCP meets with the PCP and the patient in order to address an issue of concern to both; often involves addressing a conflict between them.
- Telephone consultation: A planned, scheduled contact or follow-up with patients conducted by the BCP via telephone rather than in person.
- On-demand behavioral health or medical consultation: Usually unscheduled PCP-initiated contacts, by phone or face-to-face addressing an emergent situation requiring an immediate or short-term response by the BCP.
- Care management: Visits designed to prevent extensive and uncoordinated delivery of medical or mental health services, usually to patients

with chronic psychological and medical problems. Care management involves linking patient to a care management plan that includes multidisciplinary involvement.

- PCP consultation: A face-to-face visit with the PCP to discuss patient care issues; often involves "curbside" consultation.

Core Competencies of PCPs

- Program evaluation support: This service may involve the BCP (or practice management team) tracking PCP practices with either referred patients or populations of patients in order to assist PCPs in selecting appropriate treatments (e.g., types and dosing of medications through consistent feedback.)

According to deGruy (1999) and O'Donohue et al. (2006) the core competencies of PCPs working within an integrated care model include an understanding of the relationship between medical and psychological systems, the ability to accurately describe and promote behavioral health services when referring patients to BCP developing treatment plans that reduce physicians' visits and workloads, and effectively engaging in co-management of patient care with a BCP.

Specialty Mental Health Referral

Specialty mental health referral occurs when the primary mental health-care provider refers a patient to a mental health specialist located away from the primary care site. For example, a primary care physician may refer a patient to a therapist or a psychiatrist at a mental health clinic. A successful specialty mental health referral requires that: (1) a health-care worker recognizes that there is a problem; (2) the health-care worker needs to decide to refer rather than to treat the problem; and (3) the patient needs to show up at the referral appointment.

A successful referral has important implications for the patient since a specialist is more likely to be able to deliver care tailored to his or her specific needs. Not all mental health problems need a specialty referral, nor is this desirable for cost reasons. With older adults, however, needed referrals frequently do not occur. As mentioned earlier, untreated mental health problems account for a large percentage of primary care physician visits by the elderly. Primary care physicians detect and adequately treat or refer only 40–50% of patients with mental health problems (Speer & Schneider, 2003). Even if the physician identifies the need for a referral, older persons may resist for reasons of stigma, especially common with the current cohort of older persons, or for logistical or cost reasons, or ultimately they may simply not show up for the referral appointment.

Evidence-Based Practices for Specialty Mental Health Referral

Determining That There Is a Problem

Health-care professionals, including physicians, social workers, and nurses, frequently encounter situations in which they suspect that a patient is experiencing a psychological problem. Conditions that frequently present in the primary care setting include depression, anxiety, at-risk drinking, dementia, psychosis, mania, and hypomania. The health-care worker making the referral need not develop a specific diagnosis. A variety of assessment instruments are available to help identify problems, any one of which may be administered in the primary care environment to help inform any referral decision. Any assessment instrument should be administered and the results interpreted by persons who have received appropriate training in the proper use of the instrument.

Bartels, Coakley, Zubritsky, and PRISM-E Investigators (2004) included the following instruments in their assessment of older patients in the primary care setting:

- Review of demographic data, which may indicate areas where the patient is likely to need help. For example, the patient may have experienced a recent bereavement.
- Detailed medication review. Medication or interactions between medications can cause a variety of mental health problems, including depression and psychosis, as can a variety of common medical conditions (e.g., urinary tract infections). This is more likely to be a problem for older adults, many of whom take multiple medications.
- An alcohol quantity/frequency scale.
- The Mini-International Neuropsychiatric Interview to assess for psychosis, mania, and hypomania. It takes about 15 minutes to administer (Sheehan, Lecrubier, & Sheehan, 1998).
- Center for Epidemiological Studies Depression Scale (CES-D Scale) (Radloff, 1977).
- Beck Anxiety Inventory (Beck, Epstein, & Brown, 1988).
- The Short Michigan Alcohol Screening Test—Geriatric Version (Blow, 1991).
- The Paykel Suicide Scale to assess for suicide risk (Paykel, Myers, & Lindenthal, 1974).

- The Medical Outcomes Study 36-Item Short Form (Ware & Sherbourne, 1992) to assess for limitations in roles caused by physical or emotional problems.
- Other instruments include the Mini Mental-State Exam (MMSE), used to help assess for cognitive impairment (Folstein, Folstein, & McHugh, 1975) and the 15-item Geriatric Depression Scale (GDS15), which has been shown to be effective in screening for depression in elderly primary care attenders (D'Ath, Katona, & Mullan, 1994).

See M. E. Maruish (2000) for detailed information on a range of assessments.

Recommendations for Specialty Mental Health

Access Providers with Specialized Mental Health Expertise. It may be difficult to determine if a problem requires a referral, particularly if there are no mental health specialists available at the primary care site. Diagnosing mental health problems in older adults is especially challenging, with mental health problems presenting as increased somatic complaints and somatic sensitivity (Strosahl, 2002). It is critical to build relationships with mental health specialists, including therapists and psychiatrists. These professionals may be willing to provide training, education, and other services, in return for the possibility of referrals to their offices. Integrated care models, in which mental health specialists are co-located with and collaborate closely with primary care professionals reduce the need for specialty mental health referral and have been shown to be highly effective in addressing mental health problems in older adults (Bartels et al., 2004).

Deciding Whether to Refer or Treat. A decision to refer is based on the referring provider's assessment of his or her ability to provide adequate treatment as well as the patient's preference, and on the method of reimbursement for the referral. A physician may decide that he or she does not have the required expertise or time to treat a presenting problem and therefore refer to a therapist or a psychiatrist at a mental health clinic for a more thorough mental health evaluation. An older person may be resistant to the idea of a referral, and stigma, cost, and logistics may be obstacles; therefore a follow-through to ensure that the referral appointment is kept is important; as is weighing the potential costs and benefits of a referral with the client. Fully explaining the process to the clients so that they know exactly what to expect as well as staying involved throughout the process are also important.

Making the Referral. The strongest predictor for someone visiting his or her primary care physician and subsequently getting a specialty mental health services referral is the level of a patient's current psychological symptoms (Sorgaard, Sandanger, & Sorensen, 1999).

To overcome obstacles to the referral, select mental health clinics that tailor services to older persons, provide transportation, provide third-party payment coverage, and minimize time from referral to visit with the specialty mental health provider. This enhanced model of specialty mental health referral is discussed by Bartels, Coakley, Zubritsky, and PRISM-E Investigators (2004). It is important to develop relationships with mental health professionals who specialize in working with older adults and to start developing a knowledge base of their specific strengths and areas of expertise. Self-help groups such as Alcoholics Anonymous, faith-based organizations, and numerous volunteer organizations offer programs that address the causes of mental health problems in the elderly, and they may be included as an adjunct to professional treatment services. Additionally, an Internet search can effectively identify available local community resources.

Specialty Referral in an Integrated Mental Health Care Environment

Integrated models emphasize co-location of services and collaboration between mental health and primary care providers. Off-site specialty referral may still occur in the integrated model if on-site specialists do not have the expertise to deal with a specific case. Bartels, Coakley, Zubritsky, and PRISM-E Investigators (2004) found an integrated model to be more effective than an enhanced referral model for improving access to mental health and substance abuse services for older adults who underuse these services. With the integrated model, the logistical difficulties associated with elderly patients traveling to a different office are reduced. Also there may be less stigma associated with receiving mental health services in the primary care office. An example of an integrated care model is the PROSPECT (Prevention of Suicide in Primary Care Elderly Collaborative Trial) study, which aimed to prevent suicide in the elderly by placing depression care managers in primary care medical settings with large numbers of elderly patients. The depression care managers were psychologists and other mental health care workers, working side by side with primary care physicians (Reynolds, 2003).

Recommendations

Be aware of cultural and cohort issues. For many elderly persons there may be a stigma associated with receiving mental health services regardless of the setting. In complex cases, an off-site referral may still be needed.

EXTENDED CARE SETTINGS

Prevalence of Extended Care

There are more than 17,000 long-term care facilities in the United States serving over 1.6 million older adults (Administration on Aging, 2004). Extended care includes the medical, social, and supportive services required by people who have lost capacity for self-care because of a chronic illness or condition. It differs from acute health care in its duration and the resistance to recovery of function of the elderly requiring extended care (Administration on Aging, 2004). The cost of extended care is enormous. According to the Administration on Aging (AoA, 2005), in 2000, 23% of the estimated $1.3 trillion in health expenditures in the United States were financed by Medicare (17.3%) and Medicaid (15.6%). The rising cost of extended care and its proportion of health-care funds is alarming. Several national and state initiatives are now focused on increasing the cost-effectiveness of providing care in extended care settings.

Challenges Within Extended Care Settings

One of the central problems in extended care settings is staff turnover. According to the American Health Care Association 2002 Nursing Position Vacancy and Turnover Survey (American Health Care Association), 2003, turnover rates for certified nursing assistants (CNAs) nationally were estimated at 71%. Annual turnover for registered nurse (RN), licensed practical nurse (LPN), and director of nursing (DON) positions was about 50% across all positions. Many factors contribute to this increasingly high turnover trend. A U.S. Senate committee on Health, Education, Labor, and Pensions report cites low wages and few benefits as contributors to nurse/aide turnover (U.S. General Accounting Office, 2001). In 1999, the average hourly wage for service workers was $9.22, where nursing-home workers were making an average of $8.29.

Staff turnover is costly. Better Jobs, Better Care (2004) reviewed the literature on the economics of staffing in extended care settings and calculated that the direct cost of turnover per frontline worker is at least $2,500. Clearly, nursing homes could benefit financially from methods that would help retain nursing staff.

Cost is not the only issue when staff turnover rates are high. Quality of care is also a concern. A 2002 GAO report (U.S. General Accounting Office, 2002) examined the spending and staffing of nursing homes in Mississippi, Ohio, and Washington. In Ohio and Washington, homes that provided more nursing hours per resident day were less likely to have repeated serious or life-threatening quality problems.

Insufficient training of nursing-home staff affects both the quality of care provided and the level of stress experienced by staff. At present, federal law mandates that nursing/aide programs have at least 75 hours of training. Twenty-six states have extended their training beyond that to try to keep up with the today's nursing-home resident needs (Department of Health and Human Services, 2002).

The impact on quality of care and the financial costs of high turnover rates have forced the nursing community to look for ways to retain trained staff, including organizational and behavioral modifications to extended care facilities. Increasing nursing staff knowledge about the possible causes and consequences of behavior will also create a less stressful work environment. A report by the U.S. Department of Health and Human Services synthesizes evaluations of methods being used to try to decrease staff turnover (http://aspe.hhs.gov/daltcp/reports/insight.htm).

In the spirit of promoting a less stressful workplace, Pillemer et al. (2003) conducted a communication intervention with the staff of 20 nursing homes and the relatives of the residents in the homes. Participants in the treatment group participated in Partners in Caregiving (PIC). PIC training included parallel training in communication and conflict resolution techniques. Also, both the staff and the family of the resident met with facility administrators and discussed facility policies and procedures, and identified possible changes to the existing establishment. Results showed that the empathy in the treatment group of staff rose considerably within six months. There was also a reduction in the likelihood of staff quitting. A reduction in conflict between staff and family was noted in the case of residents with dementia. A benefit of this intervention was that 98% of participants in the program felt like they could relate what they learned in the program to experiences they had in the nursing home (Pillemer et al., 2003). More detailed information on this program can be found at http://www.blcc.cornell.edu/CAGRI/partcare.html.

A program developed by Hegeman and Hollinger-Smith (2004), "Growing Strong Roots," at the Foundation for Long Term Care (FLTC) is designed to reduce stress among long-term care staff. This program promotes enlisting more experienced CNAs to assist new CNAs in a mentor–mentee relationship. This relationship includes working on communication skills, listening skills, and conflict management. The mentee starts the program by working the same shift as the mentor. Retention of new staff in this program went from 59% to 84% three months after its introduction. Also, retention of staff who participated as mentors increased from 69% to 90%. More information regarding this program can be found at http://www.directcareclearing house.org/practices/r_pp_det.jsp?res_id=99810# and at http://www.nyahsa. org/fltc/index.cfm.

A review by Brannon, Zinn, Mor, and Davis (2002) found that having an administrative span of control was associated with low turnover rates. Self-managed work teams (SMWT) consist of 3–15 employees who manage varied aspects of their jobs. This means they not only do the hands-on work, but they also are responsible for their own scheduling, meetings, and other administrative duties. This simple change of allowing staff to participate in the decision-making process for their jobs can result in higher job satisfaction and lead to less turnover. An added benefit of this situation is that frontline workers have the knowledge necessary to improve the quality of care for residents. So far, Yeatts, Cready, Ray, DeWitt, and Queen (2004) have established teams in five nursing homes. Quantitative data are not yet published, but qualitative data have shown positive effects of SMWT.

Examples of Care Enhancement Programs

The Wellspring Model emerged from an alliance of 11 homes in Wisconsin and targeted manipulating the administrative environment to better serve the frontline workers. In this case, top management sets policies for quality, but the workers who are familiar with the residents decide how to implement the policies. The alliance of homes shares a geriatric nurse practitioner (GNP) who goes from home to home developing and conducting training from nationally recognized clinical guidelines. Those who receive this training are responsible for teaching other staff in their facility. This model includes a combination of strategies to improve quality of care and decrease staff turnover (Reinhard & Stone, 2001). For more information visit http://www.wellspringis.org/ and http://www.cmwf.org.

Several recent initiatives are attempting to change the culture of nursing homes toward an emphasis on quality of care. One example is the Learn, Empower, Achieve, and Produce (LEAP) initiative. This initiative attempts to create an "environment of purpose" for the nursing-home staff. It uses a resident-centered approach to develop qualified, effective nursing leaders and staff, uses interactive teaching methods, and rewards best behavior. A study on the effects of LEAP found that a significantly greater proportion of staff rated work empowerment, leadership effectiveness, organizational climate, job satisfaction, and work effectiveness as excellent or above average at 6- and 12-month follow-up (Hollinger-Smith & Ortigara, 2004). More information on LEAP can be found at http://www.matherlifeways.com/.

Behavioral Programs Focused on Enhancing Resident Functioning

Behavioral studies have focused on educating nursing-home staff on the possible causes and consequences of resident's behavior. It is the hoped that by implementing behavioral interventions in the nursing facility, disruptive behavior displayed by residents will decrease and the facility will be a more stress free environment.

In their book entitled *Behaviors in Dementia*, Kaplan and Hoffman (1998) discuss five training models for long-term care facility staff. The training programs focus on managing aggressive behavior, education about dementia, skills for communication, empathy training, and problem solving. It is suggested that classroom instruction about behaviors and how to handle them are not enough. Case examples and role playing are useful and effective tools. Pre- and posttesting are also important components because they allow for the assessment of the training. Another indicator of training success is the number of incidents involving problem behaviors before and after training.

In 1999, Allen-Burge, Stevens, and Burgio published a review of behavioral interventions aimed at decreasing dementia-related challenging behaviors in nursing homes. Categories included interventions for behavioral excesses (i.e., disruptive vocalizations, wandering, and physical and verbal aggression) as well as interventions for behavioral deficits (i.e., excess dependency, lack of activity engagement, lack of social interaction, and lack of communication). The last section of the article presents a comprehensive program for training nursing staff in the use of behavioral management skills and a motivational system for long-term use.

Stevens et al. (1998) implemented a training program to promote the application of behavioral management skills by staff in a nursing home. This program consisted of five hours of in-service training, followed immediately by on-the-job training for nursing assistants (NAs). During the NA training, LPNs received training in on-the-job supervisory skills. An incentive system was used for the NA training, consisting of prizes: NAs who achieved an accuracy score of 80% or better had their names placed in a lottery. One name was drawn per week and the winner received a choice of four prizes. Also, NAs received a monthly feedback letter from the director of nursing.

This training program indicates that providing knowledge to NAs is just a first step to providing quality care. On-the-job training and staff management is also an important part of maintaining staff skills over time.

Burgio et al. (2002) evaluated a comprehensive behavior management skills training program for improving CNA skill performance in the nursing home. Five nursing units were assigned to formal staff management (FSM), and four units were assigned to conventional staff management (CSM; usual supervisory and control units). CNAs in all units received equivalent skills training. Consequently, a decrease in ineffective behavior strategies was found, but not a significant increase in effective behavior strategies. Some communication strategies were shown to increase significantly. Ultimately, the FSM group showed greater maintenance of skills at six-month follow-up; however, the FSM system was not successful at initially reducing the use of ineffective behavior management.

A study by Beck et al. (2002) took a somewhat different approach to managing disruptive behavior in the nursing home. One group received an ADL intervention, one a psychosocial activities (PSA) intervention, and the final intervention group received a combination of the two. The ADL intervention focused on addressing specific cognitive deficits that may impair ADL, communication strategies, and problem-oriented strategies for particular disabilities such as fine motor impairment and perseveration. The PSA intervention focused on meeting the psychosocial needs of the residents, that is, providing activities for interaction, enjoyment, and engagement. This study found an increase in positive affect for intervention groups, but did not find a decrease in disruptive behavior.

Another approach to alleviating the stress experienced by those working in extended care facilities emerges from the research of Baltes that has focused on preventing dependency in the elderly. Baltes and her colleagues have identified social and environmental conditions involved in fostering dependency in elders in long-term care facilities. These patterns are called the "dependency-support script." Baltes, Neumann, and Zank (1994) developed a training program for staff with the goal of increasing independence-supportive and decreasing dependence-supportive patterns in two nursing homes and a geriatric ward of a hospital. The first part of the program focused on knowledge of the communication skills to be used, facts on aging, and basic behavioral principles. The second part of the program focused on the transfer of knowledge. This transfer of knowledge included hands-on behavior modification by staff. Finally, behavioral measures were observed and recorded. Independence-supportive behaviors and dependence-supportive behaviors were assessed at pre- and postintervention for both control and intervention groups. One institution did not show a statistically significant difference between pre- and posttest on independence-supportive behaviors and dependence-supportive behaviors; however, the authors state that the institution effect may have been a factor in this finding.

SERVICES TO OLDER ADULTS IN RURAL COMMUNITIES

Adults over the age of 65 comprise 18% of the rural population compared to 15% within urban areas (Bellamy, Goins, & Ham, 2003). The term *double jeopardy* is used to describe the challenges of old age coupled with the disadvantages of living in a geographically remote area (Krout, 1986). Rural communities significantly lag behind urban areas in delivering adequate mental health services (Lawrence & McCulloch, 2001). The barriers associated with providing support to elderly persons with psychological problems in remote geographic locations are formidable. This section describes barriers to service delivery and highlights behavioral health programs that have been successful in providing services to older adults in rural settings.

Defining "Rural"

There are multiple and conflicting definitions of "rural." The U.S. Census Bureau defines "rural" as areas where people live outside metropolitan areas (which are comprised of a city with at least 50, 000 people or total population of 100,000 or more). In 1992 the AoA developed a definition of "rural" as (1) a central place with a combined minimum population of fewer than 50,000 people including adjacent areas and (2) an incorporated census place with fewer than 20,000 people (Bellamy et al., 2003). By the AoA definition, 75% of all counties in the United States can be considered "rural" with populations below 50,000; however, 80% of the U.S. population is considered to live in urban areas (Bellamy et al, 2003). The definition of "rural" impacts the distribution of federal funds to service programs. For the majority of studies reviewed in this chapter, "rural" was defined as it commonly is in the geriatric literature as "a small number of people living in residential environments in remote destinations away from suburbs, cities, or large urban areas" (Krout, 1994).

Barriers to Service Delivery

Lawrence and McCulloch (2001) noted several differences between rural and urban areas that contribute to barriers to service delivery in rural settings, including:

- *Stigmatization.* Rural residents express more negative views on mental illness that results in a negative stigmatization around mental health care and for those who access it.

- *Migration.* The economic gains for working-age rural residents migrating from rural to urban areas is 30% higher than if they remained in rural areas. It is because of this economic gain that the out migration of younger, working-age adults continues to happen in rural areas leaving the remainder of the population with fewer people of working age to provide service delivery.
- *Economic conditions.* Rural elders have financial resources 12–19% below those of urban counterparts, and in general are poorer. The lack of jobs in rural locations greatly limits the ability of the rural elderly to improve their economic status. In addition, there have been changes in health-care resulting in fewer rural elderly being eligible for social security and with minimal Medicare providers residing in rural areas (Bellamy et al, 2003).
- *Informal social support.* The traditional systems of family and community support have drastically declined in rural areas since younger family members have migrated to more urban areas for better work opportunities. This drastic loss of younger, healthier populations in rural communities and in systems of support such as the church leaves a vast older, dependent population.

The Rural Mental Health Work Group within the National Institute of Mental Health has also identified significant obstacles to rural service delivery:

- *Transportation.* It costs three times as much to reach a client in a small town versus one who resides in an urban location, due to geographic distance and terrain with barriers including inadequate roads, treacherous terrain, weather extremes, and vast traveling distances.
- *Recruitment and retention of professionals.* Rural residents are more likely to receive behavioral health care from nonspecialty providers since the recruitment and retention of qualified mental health providers continues to be a persistent problem in rural areas (Merwin, Goldsmith, & Manderscheid, 1995). Across professional categories, there are 7.2 times more psychiatrists, 3.9 times more psychologists, and 5 times more social workers per capita in urban versus rural areas (Lawrence & McCulloch, 2001). The lack of mental health professionals results in a poor quality of mental health care for rural residents and a dominant focus on physical rather than mental health concerns (Lawrence & McCulloch, 2001).
- *Interagency coordination.* There is a lack of collaboration in rural settings between physical and mental health care. The majority of collaborations in rural settings are centered on exchanging information, with

client referrals and sharing of resources occurring less frequently (Lawrence & McCulloch, 2001). Interagency coordination or the collaboration of mental and physical health care is an important factor in the delivery of appropriate rural mental health care (Bull, 1998).

- *Community support.* There are few data addressing community advocacy for improving the negative views of mental health and the emphasis placed on physical illness relative to psychological health by rural residents (Lawrence & McCulloch, 2001).

Models of Rural Mental Health Service Delivery

The National Resource Center for Rural Elderly initiated a national search for successful models of rural mental health delivery in 1995 and found that successful models fell into two categories: educational and direct service models (Bane & Bull, 2001). Direct service models focus on delivering the service to the person in the most successful way, while educational models focus on increasing people's knowledge on aging, mental health, and appropriate services.

Direct Service Models

Gatekeeper Models. Gatekeepers are individuals who live in the community who come into contact with rural elders in need of mental health through their regular business activities (Bane & Bull, 2001). Not surprisingly, at-risk elders in high need of mental health services do not independently seek services (Bane & Bull, 2003). Gatekeepers have been very effective in identifying isolated elders in need of care. The Spokane Elderly Care Program (Spokane, Washington) exemplifies a successful rural gatekeeper model, relying on a team of bank personnel, postal workers, meter readers, telephone personnel, and the like who come into contact with at-risk, isolated, older adults. The purpose of this program is to deliver needed in-home services to rural older adults in order to maintain them in their homes for as long as possible. The gatekeeper refers at-risk elderly to an interdisciplinary team that responds by conducting in-home evaluations and providing ongoing clinical case management. This program has been replicated by the Mental Health of the Rural Elderly Outreach Project in rural Iowa and the Psychogeriatric Rural Elderly Outreach Program in rural Virginia (Bane & Bull, 2001).

Peer Counseling. According to Bane and Bull (2001) peer counseling programs such as the Geriatric Peer Counseling program in Mount Vernon, Washingon, are successful for three reasons: (1) volunteers are trained to collaborate with mental health professionals to provide interventions; (2) a peer counselor is often a member of the elderly clients' community and has a personal understanding of the rural environment; and (3) peer counselors are less likely to have a negative stigmatization by rural older adults compared to professionals.

Behind most rural direct service models, there is a committed individual who organized and began mental health service delivery for the community resulting in a program accessible to rural clients. The mental health program was easily accessible to clients across the rural area, and allowed clients the flexibility to use services they found most useful or effective for them.

Educational Models

In 1993 the AoA funded the development of three educational models with the goals of training nonprofessionals in recognizing mental health issues in rural older adults and in making appropriate referrals (Bane & Bull, 2001). The priority of these projects was to increase the understanding of mental health needs of rural older adults and the development of effective mental collaboration with mental health providers.

Arizona, Mental Health. This educational program targeted Latinos, Caucasians, and Native Americans through educational workshops for rural families, the general public, and non–mental health staff on the areas of mental health symptoms, effective behavior management with older adults suffering from psychiatric conditions, and appropriate referral of clients to appropriate mental health services.

Missouri, Mental Health and Aging. The purpose of this project was to educate service providers on mental health issues of rural elderly, identification of rural elderly in need of mental health services, improvement of providers' ability to inform elderly clients of services, referral of clients, and improvement of providers' ability to inform agencies of potential clients.

Project A.W.A.R.E, Pennsylvania. This project employs a cross-system model of training, including focus groups and the training of nonprofessional community caregivers, volunteers, and gatekeepers to deliver educational programs to the community. The cross-system model brought personnel together from mental health and aging systems at meetings, and also involved developing a training manual with guidelines on how to train nonprofessionals on mental health and aging issues.

The inclusion of community leaders was crucial to the success of the programs. Successful educational programs included focus groups or committees with rural community leaders in the groups, committees that developed specialized curriculums for specifically rural elderly, and committees that advertised their program to the surrounding community and recruited participants.

State and Local Initiatives on Rural Mental Health in the Elderly

In 1989, The National Resource Center for Rural Elderly (NRCRE) collected data from states regarding their initiatives in rural mental health and found that meeting the mental health needs of the rural elderly was rarely a priority for states even if it was noted that the rural elderly were in significant need of mental health services (Bane, Rathbone-McCuan, & Galliher, 1994). The data collected from the NRCRE also found that there were few programs that addressed the issue of mental health of rural older adults. A review of successful characteristics of service programs for the elderly was included in "Mental Health Services for the Elderly in Rural America" (Bane et al., 1994). Key components of success include:

- Case management tailored to fit the needs of the target population and able to fulfill the service demands of the area.
- Coalitions formed to bring resources together to meet the needs of underserved adult populations at risk for institutionalization.
- A written interorganizational agreement between involved agencies clarifying the separate and coordinated responsibilities of the different agencies.
- Identification of the mental health agency to be the lead service agency to plan and monitor the delivery of services.
- The use of communication technology to reduce the effect of distance between clients and professionals.
- Attention to problems related to alcoholism and prescription drug use.
- Consumer-friendly community education on mental health services.

State programs that embodied the preceding characteristics can serve as models for future programs (Bane et al., 1994). Some examples include:

- *Ohio Department of Aging.* This program developed an integrated social service model using coordinated case management that brought together informal and formal networks to meet the mental health needs of older adults in a rural area.

- *Indiana Department of Human Services, Division of Aging Services*. A program entitled Community and Home Options to Institutional Care for Elderly and Disabled (CHOICE) was developed to help physically frail older adults and was expanded to service mental health needs as psychiatric problems were identified as risk factors promoting disability in the elderly.
- *Eastern Oregon Human Services Consortium in La Grande*. This program used telecommunication via two-way satellite to consult with rural primary care physicians and mental health providers in rural areas. Mental health professionals were available through telecommunication from the Eastern Oregon Psychiatric center to provide case management with rural providers.
- *Abbe Center for Community Mental Health of Cedar Rapids, Iowa*. In cooperation with the Heritage Agency on Aging, an outreach program was developed to service rural elderly with psychosocial screenings held at churches, elderly clinics, and various other community settings. Referrals are made by gatekeepers in the community to a multidisciplinary team consisting of a psychiatrist, nurse, nurse practitioner, and a social worker conducting in-home evaluations along with follow-up treatment plans.

In all of the successful models of rural mental health service delivery, collaboration among mental health and other aging service providers was a key part of the program. State level initiatives that create collaboration between units of aging and departments of mental health are a necessary step to more effective service delivery to rural older adults (Bane et al., 1994).

FURTHER READING

Faith-Based Programs

Jewell, A. (Ed.). (1999). *Spirituality and ageing* (pp. 14–19). London: Jessica Kingsley Publishers Ltd.

MacKinlay, E. (2001). *The spiritual dimension of ageing*. London: Jessica Kingsley Publishers Ltd.

Related Websites

The Roundtable on Religion and Social Welfare Policy (www.religionandsocialpolicy.org) conducts in-depth, nonpartisan research to fill broad gaps in knowledge about the effectiveness and capacity of faith-based social services, policy, and regulatory changes affecting their work, and the constitutional issues involved in public funding.

CAPPE/ACPEP—The Canadian Association for Pastoral Practice and Education (www.cappe.org) is concerned with a holistic approach to health care and personal development with a special focus on spiritual and religious care.

Primary Care

James, L. C., & Folen, R. A. (2005). *The primary care consultant.* Washington, DC: American Psychological Association.

Cummings, N. A., O'Donohue, W. T., & Ferguson, K. E. (2003). *Behavioral health as primary care: Beyond efficacy to effectiveness.* Reno, NV: Context Press.

Maruish, M. E. (2000). *Handbook of psychological assessment in primary care settings.* Mahwah, NJ: Lawrence Erlbaum Associates, Inc.

Related Web Sites

www.behavioral-health-integration.com, web site of Mountain View Consulting Group, a company specializing in behavioral health integration.

www.prochange.com, web site of Pro-Change, a behavior change management company.

Extended Care

Molinari, V. (2000). *Professional psychology in long term care: A comprehensive guide.* New York: Hatherleigh Press.

REFERENCES

Administration on Aging [AoA] (n.d.a.). Aging Internet Information Notes—Health and Long Term Costs and the Elderly. Retrieved February 12, 2006, from http://www.aoa.gov/prof/notes/Docs/Health_Long_Term_Care_Costs.pdf.

Administration on Aging [AoA] (n.d.b.). Aging Internet Information Notes—Nursing Homes. Retrieved February 12, 2006, from http://www.aoa.gov/prof/notes/Docs/Nursing_Homes.pdf.

Aitken, J. B., & Curtis, R. (2004). Integrated health care: Improving client care while providing opportunities for mental health counselors. *Journal of Mental Health Counseling, 26,* 321–331.

Allen-Burge, R., Stevens, A. B., & Burgio, L. D. (1999). Effective behavioral interventions for decreasing dementia-related challenging behavior in nursing homes. *International Journal of Geriatric Psychiatry, 14,* 213–232.

American Association of Suicidology (2002). *Fact sheet: Suicide and the elderly*. Retrieved November 19, 2004, from http://www.211begbend.org/hotlines/suicide/suicidandtheelderly.pdf.

American Health Care Association. (2003). *Results of the 2002 AHCA Survey of Nursing Staff Vacancy and Turnover in Nursing Homes*. Retrieved January 20, 2005, from http://www.ahca.org/research/rpt_vts2002_final.pdf.

Baltes, M. A., Neumann E. M., & Zank, S. (1994). Maintenance and rehabilitation of independence in old age: An intervention program for staff. *Psychology and Aging, 9,* 179–188.

Bane, D. S., Rathbone-McCuan, E., & Galliher, J. M. (1994). *Mental health services for the elderly in rural America. Providing community-based services to the rural elderly*. Thousand Oaks, CA: Sage Publications, Inc.

Bane, S. D., & Bull, C. N. (2001). Innovative rural mental health service delivery for rural elders. *Journal of Applied Gerontology, 20,* 230–240.

Bartels, S. J., Coakley, E. H., Zubritsky, C., & PRISM-E Investigators. (2004). Improving access to geriatric mental health services: A randomized trial comparing treatment engagement with integrated versus enhanced referral care for depression, anxiety, and at-risk alcohol use. *American Journal of Psychiatry, 161*(8), 1455–1462.

Beck, A. T., Epstein, N., & Brown, G. (1988). An inventory for measuring clinical anxiety: Psychometric properties. *Journal of Consulting & Clinical Psychology, 56*(6), 893–897.

Beck, C. K., Vogelpohl, T. S., Rasin, J. H., Uriri, J. T. O'Sullivan, P., Walls, R., et al. (2002). Effects of behavioral interventions on disruptive behavior and affect in demented nursing home residents. *Nursing Research, 51,* 219–228.

Bellamy, G. R., Goins, R. T., & Ham, R. J. (2003) Overview: Definitions, clinical issues, demographics, health care, and long term care. In *Best practices in service delivery to the rural elderly*. Report from the West Virginia University Center on Aging.

Benjamins, M. R. (2004). Religion and functional health among the elderly: Is there a relationship and is it constant? *Journal of Aging and Health, 16*(3), 355–374.

Better Jobs Better Care. (2004). *The cost of frontline turnover in long-term care*. Retrieved January 21, 2005, from http://www.bjbc.org/content/docs/TCCost Report.pdf.

Blow, F. C. (1991). Short Michigan Alcoholism Screening Test—Geriatric Version (SMAST-G). Ann Arbor, MI: University of Michigan Alcohol Research Center.

Brannon, D., Zinn, J., Mor, V., & Davis, J. (2002). Exploration of job, organizational and environmental factors associated with high and low nursing assistant turnover. *Gerontologist, 42*(2), 159–168.

Bull, C. N. (1998). Aging in rural communities. *National Forum, 78,* 38–41.

Burgio, L. D., & Stevens, A. B. (1999), Behavioral interventions and motivational systems in the nursing home. In R. Schulz, G. Maddox and M. P. Lawton (Eds.), *Annual review of gerontology and geriatrics* (pp. 284–320). New York: Springer Publishing.

Burgio, L. D., Stevens, A. B., Burgio, K. L., Roth, D. L., Paul, P., & Gerstle, J. (2002). Teaching and maintaining behavior management skills in the nursing home. *Gerontologist, 42,* 487–496.

Chambless, D. L., & Hollon, S. D. (1998). Defining empirically supported therapies. *Journal of Clinical and Consulting Psychology, 66*(1), 7–18.

Conwell, Y. (1997). Management of suicidal behavior in the elderly. *Psychiatric Clinics of North America, 20*(3), 667–683.

Coyle, B. R. (2001). Twelve myths of religion and psychiatry: Lessons for training psychiatrists in spiritually sensitive treatments. *Mental Health, Religion & Culture, 4*(2), 149–174.

Cummings, N. A. (1997). Pioneering integrated systems: Lessons learned, forgotten, and relearned. In N. A. Cummings, J. L. Cummings & J. N. Johnson (Eds.), *Behavioral health in primary care: A guide for clinical integration* (pp. 23–35). Madison, CT: Psychosocial Press.

D'Ath, P., Katona, P., & Mullan, E. (1994). Screening detection and management of depression in elderly primary care attenders: 1. The acceptability and performance of the 15 item Geriatric Depression Scale (GDS15) and the development of short versions. *Family Practice, 11*(3), 260–266.

deGruy, F. V. (1999). The primary care provider's view. In R. R. Goetz, D. A. Pollack & D. L. Cutler (Eds.), *Advancing mental health and primary care collaboration in the public sector* (pp. 33–39). San Francisco: Jossey-Bass.

Department of Health and Human Services, Office of Inspector General. (2002). *Nurse aid training.* (Publication No. OEI-05-01-00030). Retrieved January 20, 2005, from http://oig.hhs.gov/oei/reports/oei-05-01-00030.pdf

Druss, B. G., Rohrbaugh, R. M., & Levinson, C. M. (2001). Integrated medical care for patients with serious psychiatric illness. *Archives of General Psychiatry, 58,* 861–868.

Folstein, M. F., Folstein, S. E., & McHugh, P. R. (1975). A practical method for grading the cognitive state of patients for the clinician. *Journal of Psychiatric Research, 12,* 189–198.

Fries, J., Koop, C., & Beadle, C. (1993). Reducing health care costs by reducing the need and demand for medical services. *The New England Journal of Medicine, 329,* 321–325.

Gallo, J. J., Zubritsky, C., Maxwell, J., & PRISM-E Investigators. (2004). Primary care clinicians evaluate integrated and referral models of behavioral health care for older adults: Results from a multisite effectiveness trial (PRISM-E). *Annals of Family Medicine, 2,* 305–309.

Harrison, M. O., Koenig, H. G., & Hays, J. C. (2001). The epidemiology of religious coping: A review of recent literature. *International Review of Psychiatry, 13*(2), 86–93.

Hayes, S. C., Barlow, D. H., & Helson-Gray, R. O. (1999). *The scientist practioner: Research and accountability in the age of managed care.* Needham Heights, MA: Allyn & Bacon.

Hegeman, C., & Hollinger-Smith, L. (2004). *Growing strong roots and project LEAP for a 21st century long-term care workforce: Improving staff retention and quality.* Symposium conducted at the Joint Conference of the National Council on Aging and the American Society on Aging, San Francisco, CA.

Helm, H. M., Hays, J. C., & Flint, E. P. (2000). Does private religious activity prolong survival? A six-year follow-up study of 3,851 older adults. *Journals of Gerontology: Series A: Biological Sciences & Medical Sciences, 55A*(7), M400–M405.

Holinger-Smith, L., & Ortigara, A. (2004). Changing culture: Creating a long-term impact for a quality long-term care workforce. *Alzheimer's Care Quarterly, 5*(1), 60–70.

Humphreys, K., Wing, S., & McCarty, D. (2004). Self-help organizations for alcohol and drug problems: Toward evidence-based practice and policy. *Journal of Substance Abuse Treatment, 26*(3), 151–158.

Kaplan, M., & Hoffman, B., (Eds.) (1998). *Behaviors in dementia.* Baltimore, MD: Health Professions Press.

Kaplan, M. S., Adamek, M. E., & Martin, J. L. (2001). Confidence of primary care physicians in assessing the suicidality of geriatric patients, *International Journal of Geriatric Psychiatry, 16*(7), 728–734.

Kessler, R. C., Mickelson, K. D., & Zhao, S. (1997). Patterns and correlates of self-help group membership in the United States. *Social Policy, 27,* 27–46.

Kirchner, J. E., Cody, M., & Thrush, C. R. (2004). Identifying factors critical to implementation of integrated mental health services in rural VA community-based outpatient clinics. *Journal of Behavioral Health Services & Research, 31,* 13–25.

Kodner, D. L., & Kyriacou, C. K. (2003). Bringing managed care home to people with chronic, disabling conditions: Prospects and challenges for policy, practice, and research. *Journal of Aging and Health, 1.5, Special issue: From Philosophy to Practice: Selected Issues in Financing and Coordinating Long-Term Care,* 189–222.

Krout, J. A. (1986). *The aged in rural America.* Westport, CT: Greenwood Press.

Krout, J. A. (1994). *An overview of older rural populations and community based services. Providing community-based services to the rural elderly.* Thousand Oaks, CA: Sage Publications, Inc.

Lawrence, S. A., & McCulloch, J. B. (2001) Rural mental health and elders: historical inequities. *The Journal of Applied Gerontology, 20,* 144–169.

Maruish, M. E. (2000). *Handbook of psychological assessment in primary care settings.* Mahwah, NJ: Lawrence Erlbaum Associates.

Mauer, B. J. (2003, May). *Background paper: Behavioral health/primary care integration models, competencies, and infrastructure.* Retrieved January 16, 2005, from the National Council for Community Behavioral Healthcare Web site: http://www.nccbh.org/SERVICE/consult/consult-pdf/PrimaryCareDiscPaper.pdf.

McCullough, M. E., Hoyt, W. T., & Larson, D. B. (2000). Religious involvement and mortality: A meta-analytic review. *Health Psychology, 19*(3), 211–222.

Merwin, E. I., Goldsmith, H. F., & Manderscheid, R. W. (1995). Human resource issues in rural mental health services. *Community Mental Health Journal, 31,* 525–537.

Nightingale, F. (1860). *Notes on nursing.* London: Harrison.

O'Donohue, W., Cummings, N., Cucciare, M. A., Runyan, T., & Cummings, J. (2006). *Integrated behavioral healthcare: A guide to effective intervention.* Amherst, NY: Humanity Books.

Paykel, E. S., Myers, J. K., & Lindenthal, J. J. (1974). Suicidal feelings in the general population: A prevalence study. *British Journal of Psychiatry, 124,* 460–469.

Peterson, J., Atwood, J. R., & Yates, B. (2002). Key elements for church-based health promotion programs: Outcome-based literature review. *Public Health Nursing, 19*(6), 401–411.

Pillemer, K., Suitor, J. J., Henderson, C. R., Meador, R., Schultz, L., Robison, J., et al. (2003). A cooperative communication intervention for nursing home staff and family members of residents. *Gerontologist, 43*(II), 96–106.

Primary Behavioral Healthcare Services Practice Manual 2.0. (2002). United States Air Force, Population Health Support Division. San Antonio, TX: Brooks Air Force Base.

Radloff, L. S. (1977). The CES-D Scale: A self-report depression scale for research in the general population. *Applied Psychological Measurement, 1*(3), 385–401.

Reinhard, S., & Stone, R. (2001). The Commonwealth Fund. *Promoting quality in nursing homes: The Wellspring model.* Retrieved February 10, 2005, from http://www.cmwf.org.

Reynolds, C. F. (2003). Meeting the mental health needs of older adults in primary care: How do we get the job done? *Clinical Psychology: Science & Practice, 10*(1), 109–111.

Sheehan, D. V., Lecrubier, Y., & Sheehan, K. H. (1998). The Mini-International Neuropsychiatric Interview (M.I.N.I): The development and validation of a structured diagnostic psychiatric interview for DSM-IV and ICD-10. *Journal of Clinical Psychiatry, 59*(Suppl. 20), pp. 22–33.

Simon, G. E., & Vonkorff, M. (1997). Is the integration of behavioral health into primary care worth the effort? A review of the evidence. In N. A. Cummings, J. L. Cummings & J. N. Johnson (Eds.), *Behavioral health in primary care: A guide for clinical integration* (pp. 145–161). Madison, CT: Psychosocial Press.

Sink, K. M., Holden, K. F., & Yaffe, K. (2005). Pharmacological treatment of neuropsychiatric symptoms of dementia: A review of the evidence. *Journal of the American Medical Association, 293,* 596–608.

Slay, J. D., & McLeod, C. (1997). Evolving an integration model: The 'Healthcare Partners' experience. In N. A. Cummings, J. L. Cummings & J. N. Johnson (Eds.), *Behavioral health in primary care: A guide for clinical integration* (pp. 121–141). Madison, CT: Psychosocial Press.

Sorgaard, K. W., Sandanger, I., & Sorensen, T. (1999). Mental disorders and referrals to mental health specialists by general practitioners. *Social Psychiatry & Psychiatric Epidemiology, 34*(3), 128–135.

Speer, D. C., & Schneider, M. G. (2003). Mental health needs of older adults and primary care: Opportunity for interdisciplinary geriatric team practice. *Clinical Psychology: Science & Practice, 10*(1), 85–101.

Stevens, A. B., Burgio, L. D., Bailey, E., Burgio, K. L., Paul, P., Capilouto, E., et al. (1998). Teaching and maintaining behavior management skills with nursing assistants in a nursing home. *Gerontologist, 38,* 379–384.

Strawbridge, W. J., Shema, S. J., & Cohen, R. D. (2001). Religious attendance increases survival by improving and maintaining good health behaviors, mental health, and social relationships. *Annals of Behavioral Medicine, 23*(1), 68–74.

Strosahl, K., Baker, N. J., & Braddick, M. (1997). Integration of behavioral health and primary care services: The Group Health Cooperative model. In N. A. Cummings, J. L. Cummings & J. N. Johnson (Eds.), *Behavioral health in primary care: A guide for clinical integration* (pp. 61–86). Madison, CT: Psychosocial Press.

Strosahl, K. (1998). Integrating behavioral health and primary care services: The primary mental health care model. In A. Blount (Ed.), *Integrated primary care: The future of medical and mental health collaboration* (pp. 139–166). New York: W. W. Norton & Co., Inc.

Strosahl, K. (2002). Identifying and capitalizing on the economic benefits of primary behavioral health care. In N. A. Cummings, W. T. O'Donohue & K. E. Ferguson (Eds.), *The impact of medical cost offset on practice and research* (pp. 57–89). Reno, NV: Context Press.

U.S. General Accounting Office. (2001). *Recruitment and retention of nurses and nurse aides is a growing concern* (Publication No. GAO-01-750T). Retrieved January 20, 2005, from http://www.gao.gov/new.items/d01750t.pdf.

U.S. General Accounting Office. (2002). *Nursing homes: Quality of care more related to staffing than spending* (Publication No. GAO-02-431R). Retrieved January 21, 2005, from http://www.gao.gov/new.items/d02431r.pdf.

Unützer, J., Katon, W., & Callahan, C. M. (2002). Collaborative care management of late-life depression in the primary care setting: A randomized controlled trial. JAMA: *Journal of the American Medical Association, 288,* 2836–2845.

Ware, J. E., & Sherbourne, C. D. (1992). The MOS 36-item short-form health survey (SF-36): I. Conceptual framework and item selection. *Medical Care, 30*(6), 473–483.

Yeatts, D. E., Cready, C., Ray, B., DeWitt, A., & Queen, C. (2004). Self-managed work teams in nursing homes: Implementing and empowering nurse aid teams. *Gerontologist, 44*(2), 256–261.

Zinnbauer, B. J., & Pargament, K. I. (2000). Working with the sacred: Four approaches to religious and spiritual issues in counseling. *Journal of Counseling & Development, 78*(2), 162–171.

CHAPTER 9

Moving Toward Sustainable Services

Dean D. Krahn and Sue E. Levkoff

A critical aspect of any performance improvement process that involves implementing an evidence-based practice (EBP) is sustaining the cost-effectiveness of the changed practices. While seemingly obvious, it is frequently the case that organizations focus on cost and amount of a service delivered, but do not measure the actual effectiveness of the EBP. Those EBPs that prove to be cost-ineffective should be revised or terminated after a reasonable test period. Often, administrators terminate programs before they mature to the point that cost-effectiveness, is likely or maintain programs because they were started for political rather than for clinical reasons. In this chapter, we explore the definitions of the factors that lead to sustained changes, review a case history of the implementation of a culturally competent program for the care of elderly Hmong refugees to illustrate how sustainability factors operate in the real world, and conclude with recommendations for improving sustainability in new programs.

SHOULD A PROGRAM BE SUSTAINED?

Depending on their own perspectives and roles in the health-care system, researchers, clinicians, managers, and other change leaders will define sustainability and sustained change differently. The first step in determining whether a new program should be sustained is verifying the cost-effectiveness of the change. Consider, for instance, the perspectives of three different health-care change leaders who could be involved in improving mental health care in the same community. An expert in population health might focus on the sustained improvement of a specific health outcome measure such as decreasing the number of completed or attempted suicides in a city or state by altering emergency services for a given cost. A leader of a health-care delivery system might focus on a measure of a health service delivery process that is thought to be a good proxy for the desired health outcome. This leader might focus on timely care for newly diagnosed depression or frequency with which screens for suicidal ideation are completed in various health-care venues. Again, each of these changes would be weighed against the cost of the change. In contrast, managers of smaller programs with high demand for services often focus on sustaining funding for a program as opposed to its effectiveness. The measures here often become the number of dollars in the budget, number of patients treated, and the number of staff.

We believe that a sole focus on any one of these measures will not provide adequate information regarding sustainability. A focus only on a population health measure without a clear understanding of the budget and workforce required to achieve it is not sustainable. Conversely, a focus on budget growth or maintenance and staff recruitment or retention without a meaningful mission becomes empty, unsuccessful, and, eventually, unfunded. The best outcome measures for a program involve measures of a *population's health*, of the *process of care or service*, and of *budget and staff retention*.

WHAT MAKES CHANGE MORE LIKELY TO BE SUSTAINED?

Sustained change is more likely in an organization in which planning for sustainable change is part of the mind-set and culture. That type of organization would only make a change or implement an EBP if it was judged (a) likely to improve one of the consumer mental health outcomes that represented a core part of their organizational mission; (b) able to be integrated into the organization's health care delivery processes in a manner that was practical and doable; and (c) likely to be supportable within predicted budget, staff, and space supplies. We encourage organizations to stretch their missions, reorganize their processes, and grow their resources, but only with some clear forethought about the implications of these changes. This forethought and planning should help ensure that new programs or EBPs will not damage other programs in the organization by commanding too many resources and negatively affecting the entire organizational environment. Shediac-Rizkallah and Bone (1998) listed three reasons to aim for program sustainability: (1) when the negative health outcome that was the original motivation for the new program still exists (assuring the new program has evidenced at least some success); (2) when many programs are discontinued (i.e., have poor sustainability) due to funding withdrawal after the expenditure of start-up costs, but before the new activities have reached full fruition; and (3) when a repeated failure to sustain programs not only sours the environment for performance improvement within the organization, but also within the communities of consumers and funding agencies.

DEFINING SUSTAINABILITY

Are there characteristics of new projects that predicted sustained functioning of the new program? Several research groups have attempted to identify and classify predictors of sustainability. Shediak-Rizkallah and Bone (1998), using a definition of sustainability as "program continuation," defined three groups of potentially influential factors on project sustainability, namely, project design and implementation factors, factors related to characteristics of the organization, and factors in the broader community environment:

1. Project design and implementation factors include (a) whether project goals were set with community support and involvement; (b) whether the project is perceived as successful; (c) whether the project is dependent on time-limited grant funds; (d) whether ongoing funding is available in the agency or community; (e) whether the project is preventive or treatment focused; and (f) whether education/training is part of the project.
2. Factors related to organizational characteristics include (a) whether the organization is stable and resourceful; (b) whether the project is well integrated into the organization's missions and practices; and (c) whether there is a powerful champion within the organization for the program.
3. Factors in the broader community environment include (a) whether there is a favorable socioeconomic and political environment for continuing the program in the community and (b) whether there is widespread, meaningful participation of the community in the program.

The conceptual framework of Shediac-Rizkallah and Bone formed the basis of a structured questionnaire used by Evashwick and Ory (2003) in interviews of 20 innovative, award-winning, and sustained programs defining health care and social support to the elderly. This study both operationalized the Shediak-Rizkallah and Bone conceptual model and resulted in the authors' delineating important "lessons learned." These included lessons related to each of the three broad groups of factors posited as predictors of sustainability. The first lesson is that viable, continued change is often dependent on the vision and energy of a strong leader, at least until the new program becomes embedded in the larger organization. Second, involvement of the larger community and stakeholders is considered critical by these successful programs. Third, all of these successful, sustained, innovative programs are, in fact, housed in and sponsored by an established program with resources. These resources include not only money, but also skills in implementing and sustaining new programs. Other factors that are important (and probably necessary) include active outreach, collection of outcome data, achieving financial self-sufficiency (which includes moving from soft grant money to permanent funding), maintaining a shared vision with other programs in the organization, and recognizing behavioral change principles. These two studies together resulted in the identification of a number of critical factors in programs that had made continuing or sustained changes.

A study by Gustafson et al. (2003) took a different, more rigorous approach to the identification of the factors in a Bayesian model that could predict sustained success of health-care improvement projects. Sustained success was defined as a process improvement still operating with management and staff support six months after start-up. The Gustafson-led research group used a panel of theoretical and practical experts who participated in Integrative Group Process (Gustafson, Cats-Baril, & Alemi, 1992) to identify and weight factors thought to be predictive of success as well as potentially modifiable. The group eventually agreed upon 18 factors as well as on questions that could be used to determine to what degree these factors were present in a given health-care process improvement. The 18 factors initially identified for inclusion in the model for predicting success were:

1. Exploration of problem and customer needs.
2. Change agent prestige, commitment, and customer focus.
3. Source of ideas.
4. Funding.
5. Advantages to staff and customers.
6. Radical design.
7. Flexibility of design.
8. Mandate.
9. Leader goals, involvement, and support.
10. Supporters and opponents.
11. Middle manager goals, involvement, and support.

12. Tension for change.
13. Staff needs assessment, involvement, and support.
14. Evidence of effectiveness.
15. Complexity of implementation.
16. Work environment.
17. Monitoring and feedback.
18. Required staff changes.

Finally, the size of effect of the presence or absence of a given factor was agreed upon by the group allowing creation of a Bayesian model (i.e., using common sense and real-world knowledge to eliminate needless complexity in the model). The validity and performance of the model was then assessed by comparing its predictions to the known outcomes of 221 performance improvement efforts that occurred between 1996 and 2000. These efforts as well as the outcomes (success/failure) were described by 198 senior leaders of health-care organizations. The model significantly and powerfully predicted success and failure. Further research using similar methods reported by Gustafson et al. identified change adaptability, champion status, ongoing leadership, staff motivation, and resources devoted to the change as statistically significant predictors of sustained change. Thus, the conceptual models are beginning to have an empiric footing. Those wishing to create sustainable change would do well to focus on the factors supported by data.

IMPLICATIONS OF THE LITERATURE

The preceding studies related to the sustainability of change in health care do not address improvements or EBP implementation in mental health and substance abuse programs. Yet, on the whole, the factors identified ring true to the authors who are experienced in mental health-care improvement initiatives. The first important concept is that the members of a team launching a new program must plan for sustainability from the first day of a nascent program. The second important concept is that the team seeking sustainable change must address factors at multiple levels including those factors internal to the team and its proposed EBP; those factors external to the team but within the parent organization; those factors external to the organization but within the community of interest; and, finally, those factors external to the community but still relevant. While these four levels of factors (see Figure 9.1) must be evaluated and addressed, it is likely that the team will have the most control of outcomes at the level internal to the team. It is important, however, to not be overly focused on the internal team level as factors at the

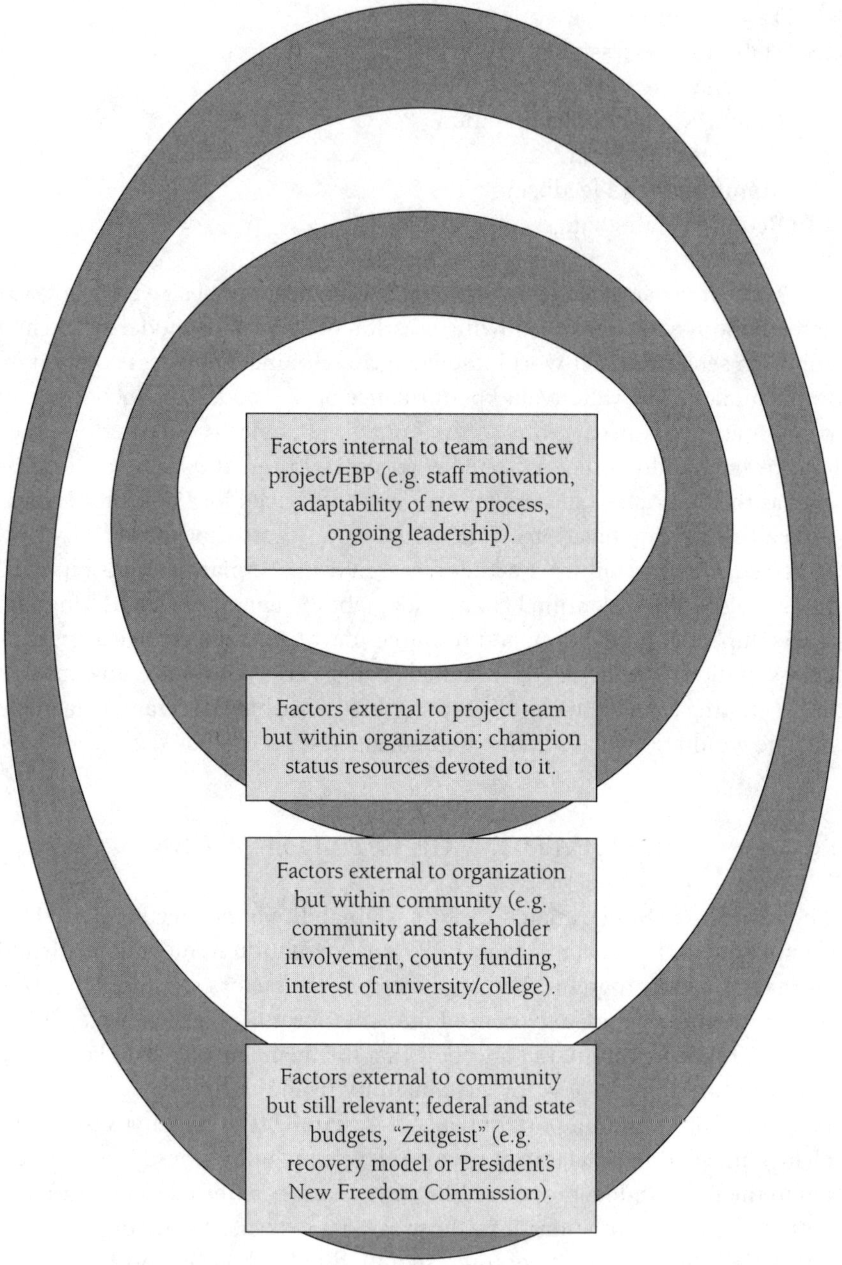

Factors internal to team and new project/EBP (e.g. staff motivation, adaptability of new process, ongoing leadership).

Factors external to project team but within organization; champion status resources devoted to it.

Factors external to organization but within community (e.g. community and stakeholder involvement, county funding, interest of university/college).

Factors external to community but still relevant; federal and state budgets, "Zeitgeist" (e.g. recovery model or President's New Freedom Commission).

FIGURE 9.1   Factors predicting sustainable change.

other levels can destroy the continuation of an excellent project. Conversely, the other levels can also help ensure success of a project by providing the resources and environment required for maturation and success.

FROM IMPLEMENTING TO SUSTAINING A PROGRAM

Factors determining the success of implementing an evidence-based program may seem similar to those guiding the program towards it sustaining performance in the long run, but a careful analysis will reveal slight but essential differences.

In a recent online publication, the Louis de la Parte Florida Mental Health Institute, University of South Florida, has performed an excellent review of the existing literature on factors determining successful implementation of an EBP (Fixsen, Naoom, Blase, Friedman, & Wallace, 2005). The review has inductively led to four basic sets of factors that are considered crucial for implementing an EBP: (1) source of the original EBP; (2) destination of the EBP; (3) communication or mechanisms to ensure fidelity and implementation quality, and (4) influences from the general environment. This perspective fits perfectly with the traditional EBP implementation projects in which there is emphasis on replicating a scientifically established intervention, and thus knowledge and skills need to be directly transferred from the research community to the service community.

Based on the observations of a dozen EBP projects that were supported by the Positive Aging Resources Center, which was a main empirical source for this book, the success of an EBP implementation depends on five general processes (see Figure 9.2):

1. Selecting the best EBP with the best fit for the target population and service staff's capability.
2. Assessing feasibility by looking not only at information on clinical effectiveness, but also further ahead at the resources for training and maintenance of the project, barriers to implementation, and the degree to which the EBP should be modified in order to be applicable to a particular setting.
3. Managing the quality of EBP implementation by developing the project team's ability to orchestrate a thoughtful process of continuous improvement of the quality.
4. Using evaluation and data resources to ensure valid and effective progress of the implementation.

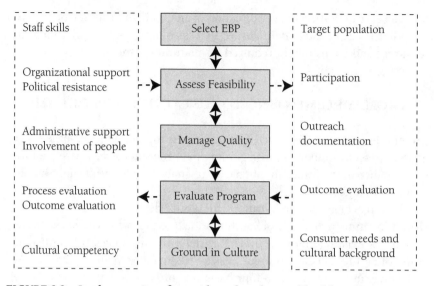

FIGURE 9.2   Implementation of an evidence-based mental health service program.

5. Integrating EBP principles with cultural characteristics of both the client population and the service providers.

These implementation processes are common among those community health centers or similar organizations that are not affiliated with academic settings, and thus have limited access to EBP resources and technical assistance. Especially if the organization provides care for medically underserved populations, such as culturally diverse groups or rural elderly people, the EBP implementation often becomes a creative integration of an EBP model and the service setting, rather than a simple execution of a guideline or protocol.

Both implementing and sustaining a program require changes in an organization that lead to desirable outcomes. They differ in their emphasis on the working processes. For successful implementation, the key word is "systematic"—systematically review the existing EBP resources and think through the target population characteristics and staff capability; systematically assess the entire organization for its readiness and barriers; systematically develop the strength of a team and capability of collecting basic data; and systematically examine the clinical flow to see how the provider behavior, treatment modality, and the general perception of the service match the culture and expectation of the target consumer groups and their community. The more thorough and careful the implementation proceeds, the higher chance for success.

Sustaining a service, in contrast, focuses on matching at fundamental levels between the new service program and its setting. First of all, the goals of the evidence-based service program should match the basic *values* and expectation of the hosting organization and community. The organization leaders need to see that the program is beneficial overall with regard to matching the mission and goals of the organization. The community needs to know, in the language that makes sense to them, that the program is successful or at least progressively promising so that it deserves the community's support. Second, the power and energy contained in an innovative service program should match the *power* structure of both the hosting organization and the receiving community. Critical elements of a program, such as its concept, leadership, and outcome data, typically carry some energy or power, but that is not enough. Program developers who care about sustainability of their programs should find at least one senior, influential manager in the organization to be so-called champion of the program. At the community level, some influential stakeholders or community leaders should be involved in the initial planning process or at least be informed of the program. Third, the developers of a sustainable EBP program should be aware of how the program *resources* and resource needs match with those of the hosting organization and community. In other words, sustainability is about what a program can bring to the organization (e.g., reputation, image, grants money, new concepts, new skills) and the community (e.g., service, leadership, thoughtful outreach programs) and how it links to what the program needs from its hosting organization (e.g., sponsorship, policy flexibility) and community (e.g., wide participation and support). Matching of value, power, and resource goes beyond the meaning of the word "adaptation." Matching entails a more active, reciprocal, and mutually respectful exchange between a functioning system and its living environment, which is the essence of sustainability.

EFFORTS TO SUSTAIN THE KAJSIAB HOUSE PROJECT

To help ourselves understand the importance of these multi-level sustainability factors (see Figure 9.2) in one of our own projects and to determine the best course of action for sustaining the Kajsiab House program for treatment and support of depressed Hmong elders, we reviewed actions taken by the program since 2003. Kajsiab House is the name not only of the program's main space (literally, *Kajsiab* House means house of "relief" or "refuge" in the Hmong language), but also of an innovative program that borrows from several EBPs including cultural competence, assertive community treatment, clubhouse, and mobile outreach approaches.

In the 1990s, more than 5,000 Hmong refugees moved to Dane County, Wisconsin, under the aegis of interested and supportive churches. When Hmong arrived in Dane County, few had language skills, job skills, or any understanding of the culture. These problems were particularly prominent among elderly Hmong (mostly women as many men in that generation had died in the long-lasting Southeast Asian wars). Faced with the language and cultural barriers of their strange new home in a strange new climate and left at home by children and grandchildren who were busy trying to survive in a new land, many elders became depressed and troubled by nightmares and flashbacks. Importantly, efforts to help the Hmong elders sprang from the recognition within the Hmong community itself that there was a terrible problem among elders who had come to the United States with their surviving family members after a harrowing life of war, killing fields, and refugee camps. This problem was recognized by the younger generations and, importantly again, a leader from the community emerged. Doua Vang not only raised the community consciousness regarding this issue but also became a clinical member of the Mental Health Center of Dane County (MHCDC), the nonprofit organization in which Kajsiab House would eventually reside. Thus, the community in some ways became part of the MHCDC and vice versa, a trend that would continue to characterize this effort. Doua Vang would become the tireless, innovative, and vital team leader. Moreover, he became an effective recruiter of other committed, younger Hmong people who would become part of Kajsiab House.

Importantly, when Doua began working at MHCDC, it was an organization that, under the leadership of two critical champions, was searching for ways to serve new, more diverse Dane County residents in a culturally competent manner. The organization as a whole had already begun a discussion on what cultural competence actually meant and how the organization could create a cultural competence that would permeate the entire system of care. The MHCDC had previously started projects to better serve Cambodian refugees as well as the growing African American community in Dane County. So, serving the Hmong elders with depression was entirely consistent with the current mission pursued by the parent organization.

It should also be noted that MHCDC had a long history of implementing innovative, even radical, approaches as it was the home to the initial assertive community treatment programs pioneered by Stein and Santos (1998). It also was an early implementer of clubhouse and mobile outreach models of care (Comprehensive Health Enhancement Support System, 2001). Therefore, it was, and is, an organization that believes itself capable of making new ideas work. In the 1990s, budgets at the county, state, and national level were also a bit better than currently as the U.S. economy was expanding rapidly.

But, the model for Kajsiab House did not develop until (1) the right Western clinicians were working with Doua Vang and similarly minded, motivated, younger Hmong people and (2) a reasonable amount of money and space were identified. In regard to the first issue, Western psychiatrists and psychologists interacted with Hmong community members long enough to understand how a program structured similarly to a village back in Laos would form a healing, holding environment in which elders would feel comfortable enough to allow treatment of their disorders. Kajsiab House emerged as the Western providers interacted with cultural brokers (bilingual Hmong clinicians) as well as consumers and their families from the Hmong community. Not only was the community involved in needs assessments, but community members and consumers were involved in councils that make most important decisions at Kajsiab House including those regarding budget and personnel. Because the community was involved in identifying needs and the initial need was for elders to again interact with other Hmong elders in a positive way, the initial focus was not on healing the patients but on letting them become a part of the community or village. So, initial outcome measures were based on attendance at Kajsiab House and participation in activities. As these traumatized elders felt ready, they chose to see the psychiatrist or psychologist and they chose whether or not to follow the advice of those who treated them. Pursuit of non-Western approaches to healing are accepted and encouraged as a sign that the elder is working to get better.

Money and space for this program developed in a way that reflects the importance of taking advantage of opportunities in the larger environments in which a proposed new program or change will exist. A financial opportunity emerged when the Wisconsin State Refugee Office along with other state agencies made money available for Kajsiab House using the argument that younger Hmong refugees would continue to find it difficult to establish regular work and income until there was a mechanism by which care could be provided for the elders. Space was available due to the empty buildings that existed at the state hospital. Thus, financial opportunities and space opportunities emerged at a time when a leader, a community, and a group of interested clinicians had reached a point that allowed them to seize those opportunities. With the development of Kajsiab House, more than 80 elders per week and their families benefit from care. The more Western care such as psychiatrist visits and group therapy is billable so that some financial stability and some independence from grant funding has developed. However, grants from Substance Abuse and Mental Health Services Administration (SAMHSA) and other agencies have been vital to making the budget work for the first seven years of Kajsiab House.

Doua and the MHCDC clinicians created a model that involved community input at every level so that members of the Hmong community and consumers sit on all major decision-making bodies in Kajsiab House. Moreover, Kajsiab House has involved the larger Dane County and Wisconsin community by including important community and political leaders on all of their boards. These leaders are invited to be present whenever journalists highlight Hmong cultural events staged at Kajsiab House. Connections with University of Wisconsin faculty are cultivated to increase grant possibilities and to create access to a student workforce. Hence, both consumers and funders feel a personal commitment to Kajsiab House that leads them to make efforts not often seen in a typical clinic.

Thus, up to this point, Kajsiab House has done at least some work at each of the four important levels of sustainability previously defined. At the level of factors internal to the team, Kajsiab House had an excellent, committed, strong leader; a very motivated staff as the cultural brokers who were both Hmong community members and providers; and a model that was adaptable to the problems to be addressed and to the larger organization. The implementation of the Kajsiab House program was helped dramatically by the fact that the MHCDC, the organization in which Kajsiab House was embedded, was (a) skilled in implementing new models of care; (b) interested in building a culturally competent environment; and (c) had champions for cultural competence at the organizational level. At the community level, Kajsiab House implementers both took advantage of and created some excellent sustainability factors. The Kajsiab House model was based on a clearly identified community need and involved the Hmong community from the first idea stages. Moreover, the idea of creating a model for care based on the village structure well known to elders from their time in Laos was an inherent winner in the Hmong community. But it was equally important for Doua Vang and his group to involve the larger, mainstream Dane County community in this project because that larger community had control of many of the resources needed for expansion of Kajsiab House. The strategy of consistently and significantly involving important Dane County and university leaders in the boards that run Kajsiab House has been successful. This strategy also creates a synergistic meeting of communities as members of the Hmong and mainstream cultures interact on these boards and at Hmong cultural events in ways that create personal connections and commitments. Finally, at the level of state and federal budgets and environments, Kajsiab House got its start by convincing funding agencies that its services to elders could help younger Hmong people go from welfare to work, a very popular message in Wisconsin in the 1990s when initial funding was sought. Kajsiab House has also successfully competed for federal funding of programs for seniors with a plan for cultural competency as its model was appropriate for the changing demographics of the United States.

Despite the care that was taken to address sustainability factors at all four critical levels, Kajsiab House is entering a period of some uncertainty. Changes in the economy have led to significant belt tightening in state and county budgets. Federal grants are running out and only some of the services provided by Kajsiab House can be billed to other payers. This is the time in which the unceasing work of Doua Vang to involve the Hmong community as well as the mainstream community is likely to pay off. It is also a time when having Kajsiab House housed within an organization that values cultural competence as one of its core values is critical. When decisions are made about which programs will be funded at the county or organizational level, these personal commitments and values will be important. Kajsiab House staff are also working hard at diversifying their sources of funding by seeking more university collaborators and more community donations.

It is also important for Kajsiab House to be able to tell a story of success after its first several years of existence. The lack of clinical measures in the Hmong language has hampered this effort a bit, but this deficiency created not only a drive to translate such measures into Hmong in a valid way, but also a motivation to tell important personal stories of Hmong elders and their experiences in life and at Kajsiab House. Their stories of trauma, resilience, and recovery are inherently meaningful and powerful even across cultural gaps. It is clear that just as working to improve quality is never complete, working on sustainability is never finished either. Sustaining Kajsiab House will require efforts to keep it closely aligned with the MHCDC's core goals and will require ongoing fundraising beyond clinical income.

TIPS FOR CREATING A PROGRAM THAT IS SUSTAINABLE

The creation of a sustainable program involves significant work at multiple levels. One of the biggest mistakes made by many is the belief that if one has a good clinical program (usually determined by providers of the services in that program), then others in the organization and community at administrative and funding levels should perceive this quality and should create the environment and funding that sustains the program. If no other message comes across in this chapter, the authors hope that the reader understands that this belief is a recipe for a very short program or change. A four-level plan is critical to building a program. If the leader of the program is primarily a clinician or researcher without much interest or skill in the worlds of budgets, administration, or politics, then that clinical or research leader must find an ally or cochampion to work at those levels. An excellent plan for a new program would involve a series of actions to be taken at each of the four levels as well as timelines that allow for the coordination of these actions. Moreover, there should be alternate plans (i.e., a Plan B and Plan C) at each level to which the program can turn if the original plan (i.e., Plan A) does not work out. Given the fact that the program has less and less control as it moves to organizational, then community, and, finally, state and national levels, the failure of one's first approaches must be anticipated so that the program can adjust if necessary. After all, programs are living entities and the one thing in life that is guaranteed is change. If one's program is not adaptable to changing environments, then extinction is guaranteed.

Even if a leader and his or her staff have a four-level plan worked out, there will probably be differing opinions about the degree of sustainability of the new planned program. Recently, an excellent new tool has become available that will allow the leader and staff to assess the factors that lead to sustainability. The Web site for the Network for the Improvement of Addiction Treatment, a program led by David Gustafson, at www.niatx.net has a mechanism that allows a leader and staff to conduct a project sustainability self-assessment. At that site, a project leader can register his or her team to allow the team members to answer ten questions anonymously and, hopefully, with brutal honesty. The questions assess how the leader and staff see their project in terms of the following ten factors: (1) staff involvement and training; (2) infrastructure to sustain the project; (3) benefits of the program beyond those to patients; (4) credibility of the projected benefits; (5) staff attitudes; (6) credibility and support of the senior leader; (7) credibility and support of the clinical leaders; (8) effectiveness of the outcomes monitoring system; (9) goodness of fit of the project with broader organizational goals; and (10) adaptability of the new process to the particular implementation.

After each staff member completes the "Sustainability Predictor," the project group receives feedback on how the staff rates the new project on each factor versus the best possible score and versus the average score on that factor based on the answers of many other teams involved with improvement projects in addictions. While this site has not been designed specifically for mental health projects, the process of answering these questions and going over the answers with a critical group in the improvement process will give the group a very good idea of where to put significant efforts to shore up project sustainability. Another tip is to read the improvement guide on sustainability for the National Health Service of the United

Kingdom, an organization aimed at making quality improvement and sustainability part of their culture, found at www.modern.nhs.uk/improvement guides (see also NHS Modernisation Agency, 2000).

There are few hard data regarding the sustainable use of EBPs specifically in mental health. Gustafson's team (Gustafson et al., 2003) is currently collecting information on the sustainability factors of a large number of programs implementing EBPs in substance abuse treatment. Two important points relevant to mental health sustainability can be made. First, in Gustafson's work, sustainable change was more likely when a clearly defined new paradigm or technology (like an EBP) was implemented. Second, however, various factions of the mental health treatment community continue to resist the use of such well-defined EBPs citing a variety of problems. The authors sense that this resistance might be higher in the mental health area than other areas of health care and therefore more work on building team consensus regarding the change might be necessary.

ONE LAST VIEW OF SUSTAINABILITY

Anyone who decides to put the word "sustainability" into a search engine these days will find many sites devoted to ecosystems, sustainable growth, or a sustainable economy. The state of Oregon Web site on this topic, http://oregonfuture.oregonstate.edu, discusses the area of overlap between economic needs, environmental needs, and community social needs as being the zone of livability or sustainability. It also suggests that any new enterprise needs to not only aim at increasing profits but also at improving the planet and improving people's lives. By analogy, the authors suggest that a new mental health improvement project must not only improve people's lives and make the budget, but also must aim to improve the environment in which the project exists. A new project should have a plan for how it will help the organization and community in which it exists learn and grow so that future projects will have a favorable soil in which to take root. There are many ways to do this, including community outreach and education programs, training current practitioners as well as students in a new technique, making sure administrators and funding source personnel have a personal connection with the project, and diffusing the project's precepts and techniques to neighboring programs and communities. In the world of improving the mental health of a community much like in our new cyber-based world, knowledge and skill are meant to be given away while trusting that each cycle of finding opportunities for improvement, learning, teaching, and sharing will lead to the next cycle of improvement for one's program and community.

EPILOGUE

Now that we have discerned important factors resulting in sustained change, we must make a final admission. Most changes should not be permanent as most improvements of today will eventually be supplanted by the even better improvements of tomorrow. While we certainly hope that our recommendations for improving sustainability of EBP implementations are helpful in creating lasting programs, we also recognize that any healthy organization will be scanning the environment for new approaches to improving the mental health of their consumers and community. So, like all natural systems, each EBP will have (if all goes well) a time to be planted and grow, a time to sustain, and a time to be the basis for a newer, better evidence-based practice.

REFERENCES

Comprehensive Health Enhancement Support System. (2001). *Paths to recovery.* University of Wisconsin Madison. Retrieved from http://chess.chsra.wisc.edu/Chess/.

Evashwick J. C., & Ory, M. (2003) Organizational characteristics of successful innovative health care programs sustained over time. *Family Community Health* 26(3), 177–193.

Fixsen, D. L., Naoom, S. F., Blase, K. A., Friedman, R. M., & Wallace, F. (2005). *Implementation research: A synthesis of the literature* (FMHI Publication #231). Tampa, FL: University of South Florida, Louis de la Parte Florida Mental Health Institute, The National Implementation Research Network.

Gustafson, D., Cats-Baril, W., & Alemi, F. (1992). *Systems to support health policy analysis.* Ann Arbor, MI: Health Administration Press.

Gustafson, D., Sainfort, F., Eichler, M., Adams, L., Bisognano, M., & Steudel, H. (2003). Developing and testing a model to predict outcomes of organizational change. *Health Services Research, 38*(2), 751–776.

NHS Modernisation Agency. (2002). *Improvement leaders' guide to sustainability and spread.* Ancient House Printing Group, Ipswich, Suffolk, UK. Retrieved from http://www.modern.nhs.uk.

Shediac-Rizkallah, M., & Bone, I. (1998). Planning for the sustainability of community-based health programs: Conceptual frameworks and future directions for research, practice and policy. *Health Education Research, 13*(1), 87–108.

Stein, L. I., & Santos, A. B. (1998). *Assertive community treatment for people with severe mental illness.* New York: W.W. Norton & Company.

Index

(Note: A page number followed by *t* indicates a table; by *f*, a figure.)

AA (Alcoholics Anonymous), 180, 191
Abbe Center for Community Mental
    Health of Cedar Rapids, Iowa, 202
Abilify (aripiprazole), 139
Access, 12, 32–33
Acculturation, 69, 87
Acetylcholinesterase inhibitors, 140
Active listening, 88
Activities of daily living (ADL), 179, 196
AD (department of administration), 49
ADEAR (Alzheimer's Disease Education
    and Referral) Center, 145
ADHD (attention-deficit hyperactivity
    disorder), 140
ADL (activities of daily living), 179, 196
Administration on Aging (AoA), 200
Administrative strategy, for quality
    management (QM), 38
Agoraphobia, 117
Akatinol, 141
Alcohol abuse, 119–121, 161. *See also*
    Substance use disorders
Alcoholics Anonymous (AA), 180, 191
Alprazolam, 113
Alzheimer's Association, 6, 140, 145,
    169, 170
Alzheimer's disease, 119, 135, 145
Alzheimer's Disease Education and
    Referral (ADEAR) Center, 145
American Academy of Neurology, 140
American Association for Geriatric
    Psychiatry, 7, 140

American Evaluation Association, 57
American Geriatrics Society, 140
American Health Care Association 2002
    Nursing Position Vacancy and
    Turnover Survey, 192
American Heart Association, 6
American Psychiatric Association, 6
American Psychological Association
    (APA), 4, 6, 106
American Society on Aging/National
    Council on the Aging, 7
Antidepressants, 104, 113
Antihistamines, 113
Antipsychotic medications, 146, 150–151
Anxiety
    anxiety-based administrative coping,
    54
    assessment of, 110–113
    basic facts about, 108, 109t, 110
    drug treatments for, 113–114
    instruments for assessing, 111t
    therapist-based treatments for,
    114–118
AoA (Administration on Aging), 200
APA (American Psychological
    Association), 4, 6
APA Task Force on Quality Indicators, 47
Aricept (donepezil), 140
Aripiprazole (Abilify), 139
Assessment
    anxiety, 110–113
    dementia, 137–139

Assessment (*cont.*)
  depressive disorders, 100, 101t–103t, 104
  fidelity, 51–52
  idiographic, 30–31, 162–163
  performance, 50–51, 50–57
  readiness, 17–21, 60
  risk, 27
  schizophrenia, 147–150
  service delivery, 161–164
  specialty mental health referral, 189–190
  substance abuse, 120–121
Assisted living project, 3, 12–13, 14
Attention-deficit hyperactivity disorder (ADHD), 140
Axon Idea Processor, 55–56

BA (behavioral activation), 105
Barriers
  to access services, 12
  to implementation of EBPs, 27–29
  to integrated care, 185–186
  political, 29
  to service delivery in rural settings, 197–199
  theoretical/principle-based, 28–29
BDI (Beck Depression Inventory), 163
Behavioral activation (BA), 105
Behavioral programs, for staff training in extended care settings, 195–197
Behavioral relaxation training, 114
Behaviors in Dementia, 195
Behavior therapy (BT), 104–105, 122, 137–138, 142–143
Belief systems, 72, 87
Bell Laboratories, 52
Benzodiazepines, 113
Beta-blockers, 113
Between-group heterogeneity, 68–69, 88
Bok, Chan, 56
Bonuses, as incentives, 49
Brainstorming, 46
BT (behavior therapy). *See* Behavior therapy (BT)
Bupropion, 104
Buspirone, 113

CAGE screening instrument, 121, 161
California Proposition 63 "Millionaire Tax," 1
Cappeller, Jack, 82
Cappeller, Virginia, 82
CAPS (*Clinician-Administered PTSD Scale*), 112
Caregiver Resource Centers, 169
Caregivers, 143–146, 144t
Case studies
  assisted living project, 3, 12–13, 14
  Health Improvement Program for the Elderly (Tucson), 79–84
  Kajsiab House, 217–221
  Tiempo de Oro (Phoenix), 75–79
Cause-and-effect diagram, 45
CBHPPs (church-based health promotion programs), 180
CBT (cognitive behavioral therapy). *See* Cognitive behavioral therapy (CBT)
Center for Epidemiological Studies Depression Scale (CES-D Scale), 189
Center for Mental Health Services, 175
Centura Life Center, 169
Certified nursing assistants (CNAs), 192, 194, 196
CES-D Scale (Center for Epidemiological Studies Depression Scale), 189
Challenging behaviors, 145, 196
Checklists, for performance assessment, 51
CHOICE (Community and Home Options to Institutional Care for Elderly and Disabled), 202
Chronic obstructive pulmonary disease (COPD), 187
Church-based health promotion programs (CBHPPs), 180
Clients
  culture of, 67, 73t, 82
  separating situational and cultural factors, 72–75
  values and preferences of, 29
Clinical judgment, 30
Clinical utility, 31–32
Clinician-Administered PTSD Scale (CAPS), 112

Clinician-rated Measures: Anxiety Disorders Interview Schedule, 111
Clonazepam, 113
Clozapine (Clozaril), 139, 150
CNAs (certified nursing assistants), 192, 194, 196
Cognex (tacrine), 140
Cognitive behavioral therapy (CBT)
    anxiety, 117
    CG EBP case study, 79–84
    dementia, 143
    depression, 104–105, 163
    schizophrenia, 151
    substance abuse, 123
Cognitive diffusion, 114
Cognitive impairment, 119
Cognitive restructuring, 114
Cognitive therapy, 151
Cohen-Mansfield Agitation Inventory, 137
Collaboration
    adaptation of interventions and, 13
    in integrated health care, 165–166
        (*See also* Co-location; Integrated care)
    managing resistance and, 43–44
    models of integrated health care, 167–171
    between quality management committee and administrative department, 49
    in rural settings, 198–199
    team building and, 39
Co-location, 165, 166–167, 191–192
Combination treatment, depression, 106
Communication, 48, 71, 88–89, 196
Community and Home Options to Institutional Care for Elderly and Disabled (CHOICE), 202
Community-based outreach programs, 166
Community engagement techniques, 75–78
Community support, in rural settings, 199
Comorbidities
    antipsychotic drugs, 151
    anxiety, 110, 116
    dementia, 136–137

depression, 100, 107
    nonparticipation in CG EBP interventions, 73–74
Component fidelity, 52
Computerized data tracking systems, 163–164
Concept mapping, 55
Conferences, 6–7
Confianza, 90
Consensus building, 39, 41–43, 42*t*
Consensus statements, 32
Consultation, 7, 50–51, 57, 165, 187
Consumers. *See* Clients
Context, 11, 12, 21
Contingent relationships, 137
Conventional staff management (CSM), 196
COPD (chronic obstructive pulmonary disease), 187
Coping, 54, 145, 151. *See also* Caregivers
Coping with Caregiving, 145
Coping with Frustration, 145
Coping with Schizophrenia: A Guide for Families, 152
Costs
    as a barrier to implementing EBPs, 22–23
    cost-benefit analysis, 23
    cost-effectiveness, 23–24, 32
    cost-offset analysis, 25
    cost-utility analysis, 24–25
    resource readiness and, 20
    sustainability and, 209–210
    of training, 26
CSM (conventional staff management), 196
Cultural Knowledge Rating Scale (CKRS), 87*f*
Culturally competent evidence-based practice (CC EBP), 93
Culturally grounded evidence-based practice (CG EBP)
    case studies, 76–78, 80–81, 81–82
    Cultural Knowledge Rating Scale (CKRS), 87*f*
    Cultural Skills Rating Scale (CSRS), 89*f*
    implementation, 84–86*f*

Culturally grounded evidence-based
    practice (CG EBP) (*cont.*)
  measuring, 86–91, 90*f*
  model, 75*f*
  multicultural context of, 73*f*, 87
  principles for designing and
    implementing, 68–75
  program experiences and outcomes,
    75–84
Cultural Skills Rating Scale (CSRS), 89*f*
Culture, 67–68, 70–71, 192, 210. *See also*
    Culturally grounded evidence-
    based practice (CG EBP)

Databases, 4, 38, 161, 163
Data collection, 70, 163–164
Dementia
  alcohol abuse and, 119
  basic facts about, 135–137
  caregiver functioning and, 143–146
  collaborative care models for, 169–170
  comorbidities and, 136–137
  ineffective assessments, 137
  medical assessments, 138–139
  psychological assessments, 137–138
  psychological treatments, 142–143
  psychotropic drugs for, 139–142
  screening for, 160–161
  Web site, 146
Deming, W. Edwards, 52
Department of administration (AD), 49
Department of human resources (HR), 49
"Dependency-support script," 196
Depression
  assessment, 104
  assessment of, 100
  basic facts about, 99–100
  CG EBP case study, 79–84
  comorbidities and, 100, 107
  instruments for assessing, 101*t*–103*t*
  intervention for, 104–108
  screening for, 160
  suicide and, 181
  Web site, 106
Descriptive process evaluation, 59–60*t*
*Diagnostic and Statistical Manual of Mental
    Disorders,* Fourth Edition (*DSM—
    IV*), 99, 108, 118, 146

Diaphragmatic breathing, 114
Diazepam, 113
Differential compliance, 107
Director of nursing (DON), 192
Discrimination, as a barrier to CG EBP
    participation, 74
Disruptive behavior, 145
Dissemination competence, 32
DON (director of nursing), 192
Donepezil (Aricept), 140, 141
Drug holidays, 153
Drugs. *See* Medications
*DSM—IV (Diagnostic and Statistical
    Manual of Mental Disorders,* Fourth
    Edition), 99, 108, 118, 146

Eastern Oregon Human Services
    Consortium, 202
EBPs (evidence-based practices). *See*
    Evidence-based practices (EBPs)
Economic issues, 23–27, 184, 192, 198.
    See also Costs
Eldercare Locator, 146
El Mirage community, 69, 72, 77
Emerging practice (EP), 1, 13
Enhanced referral model of integrated
    care, 165
EP (emerging practice), 1, 13
Ethnicity. *See* Race/ethnicity
e-TOCs (table of contents), 4
Evaluation
  identifying evaluators, 57
  for monitoring quality of EBPs, 56
  of outcome, 61–63, 62*t*
  planning for, 57–59
  of process, 59–60*t*, 61*t*
  quality management (QM) and, 38
  of research studies, 9
Evidence-based practices (EBPs)
  for anxiety in older adults (*See*
    Anxiety)
  assessing feasibility (*See* Feasibility)
  culturally grounding (*See* Culturally
    grounded evidence-based practice
    [CG EBP])
  for dementia (*See* Dementia)
  for depression in older adults (*See*
    Depression)

identifying, 1
managing quality in (*See* Quality
    management [QM])
for schizophrenia in late life (*See*
    Schizophrenia)
selecting (*See* Selection)
by service delivery process (*See*
    Service delivery)
within special settings (*See* Extended
    care; Faith-based behavioral health
    programs; Primary Care; Rural
    settings)
for substance use in older adults (*See*
    Substance use disorders)
sustainability of (*See* Sustainability)
Executives, readiness for change, 18–19
Exelon (rivastigmine), 140
Exposure-based interventions, 115
Extended care, 192–197. *See also*
    Assisted living project

Faith-based behavioral health programs,
    179–181, 191, 202–203
FDA (Federal Drug Administration),
    139, 140
Feasibility
    clinical utility, 31–32
    costs, 22–27
    maintaining awareness of new EBPs,
        32–33
    modification and implementation,
        27–32
    organizational climate, 21–22
    readiness assessment, 17–21
    selecting an EBP and, 11–12
Federal Drug Administration (FDA),
    139, 140
The Feeling Good Handbook (Burns), 106
Feeling Good: The New Mood Therapy
    (Burns), 106
Fidelity assessment, 51–52
Finances. *See* Costs
Fishbone diagrams, 45*t*–46, 55
Florida Coalition on Mental Health and
    Aging, 7
Flowcharts, 44–45, 53
FLTC (Foundation for Long Term
    Care), 193–194

Focus groups, 22, 82
Formal staff management (FSM), 196
Foundation for Long Term Care
    (FLTC), 193–194
FSM (formal staff management), 196

Galantamine (Reminyl), 140, 141
Gap analysis, 20
Gatekeepers, 199
GDS (Geriatric Depression Scale), 83,
    160–161, 162, 190
Gender, 99–100, 118, 136, 151
Generalizability, 9, 32
Generalized anxiety disorder, 116–117
Geodon (ziprasidone), 139
Geriatric Depression Scale (GDS), 83,
    160–161, 162, 190
Geriatric nurse practitioner (GNP), 194
Geriatric Peer Counseling program
    (Washington State), 199–200
Gerontological Society of America, 7
Get Them on Your Side (Bacharach), 43
GNP (geriatric nurse practitioner), 194
Goals readiness, 20
GPRA (Government Performance and
    Reporting Act) instrument, 79
Great-leader model, 37–38
Group Health Cooperative (Seattle),
    167, 185
Growing Strong Roots (Foundation for
    Long Term Care), 193–194
Guadalupe community, 69, 72, 77
Guidelines, 5, 32

Haloperidol, 150
Hamilton Anxiety Rating Scale, 111
Hamilton community, 69
*Handbook of Assessment in Clinical
    Gerontology,* 162
Healthcare Partners in Los Angeles
    County, 185
Health Improvement Program for the
    Elderly (Tucson)
    applying the CG EBP model, 79–84
    between-group differences and, 68
    comorbidities and program
        participation, 74
    data collection, 70

Health Improvement Program for the
    Elderly (Tucson) (*cont.*)
  relational ties, 71
  values and belief systems, 72
  within-group differences and, 68
Health literacy, 73
Heritage Agency on Aging (Iowa), 202
Heterogeneity, between- and within-
    group, 68–69
Heuristic process evaluation, 59–60, 61*t*
Hmong community. *See* Kajsiab House
Home visits, as a community
    engagement technique, 76, 79
HR (department of human resources),
    49

Idiographic assessment, 30–31, 162–163
Illiteracy, 73
IMPACT (Improving Mood-Promoting
    Access to Collaborative Treatment),
    6, 167–168
Implementation
  barriers to, 27–28
  CG EBPs, 70, 84–86*f*
  definition of, 17
  of integrated care, 186–188
  modification and, 27–32
Improving Mood-Promoting Access to
    Collaborative Treatment
    (IMPACT), 6, 167–168
Incentives, 21–22, 49
Income. *See* Socioeconomic status
Indicator of communication, 48
Information dissemination, 33
Innovation-values fit, 21, 22
Input costs, 25
Institute for Healthcare Improvement,
    52
Integrated care
  advantages of, 184
  barriers to, 185–186
  case examples of, 185
  co-location, 165, 166–167, 191–192
  comparison with current health-care
    system, 183*t*
  core competencies of primary care
    providers, 188
  implementation of, 186–188

overview, 182–183
  service delivery and, 164–166
  specialty mental health referral,
    188–191
Integrative Group Process, 212
International Psychogeriatric
    Association, 6
Interpersonal therapy (IPT), for
    treatment of depression, 104,
    105–106
Ishikawa, Kaoru, 46

Jargon, 32

Kaiser Permanente, 161, 185
Kajsiab House, 217–221
Keywords, 4–5
Knowledge readiness, 19
Korsakoff's syndrome, 119

Language, 32, 71
Law of thirds, 148
Leadership, 37–38, 43, 212, 222
LEAP (Learn, Empower, Achieve, and
    Produce), 194–195
Lewy body disease, 135, 140
Libraries, 4
Licensed practical nurse (LPN), 192
Life Satisfaction Index (LSI), 79
Literacy, 73
Literature reviews, 4, 215
Literature searches, 5–8*t*
Logic model, 58–59
Logic of evaluation, 57–58
Long-term care. *See* Extended care
Lorazepam, 113
Louis de la Parte Florida Mental Health
    Institute, 215
LPN (licensed practical nurse), 192, 195
LSI (Life Satisfaction Index), 79

MacArthur Depression in Primary Care
    Tool Kit, 5
Major depression, 99
Major depressive disorder (MDD), 9
Management. *See* Quality management
    (QM)
Manuals, 5, 32

MAOIs (monoamine oxidase inhibitors), 104
Marana Valley, 69, 80–83
MAS (Motivation Assessment Scale), 137
MDD (major depressive disorder), 9
Measurement, CG EBPs, 84–86*f*, 87*f*, 89*f*
Medical Outcomes Study 36-Item Short Form, 190
Medications. *See also specific drugs*
  antipsychotic, 146, 150–151
  benzodiazepines, 113
  gender and, 121
  psychotropic, 139–142, 184
  response to, 106
  tricyclic antidepressants, 104
Meditation, 114
Medline, 4
Memantine, 141
Mental Health Center of Dane County (MHCDC), 218
Mental Health of the Rural Elderly Outreach Project (Iowa), 199
Mental health services. *See also specific interventions*
  co-location of services and collaboration between mental health and primary care providers, 191–192
  effectiveness of primary care for mental health problems, 181–182
  specialty mental health referral, 188–191
MHCDC (Mental Health Center of Dane County), 218
Migration, rural-urban, 198
Mind-set. *See* Culture
Mini-International Neuropsychiatric Interview, 189
Mini Mental-State Exam (MMSE), 190
Minnesota Multi-phasic Personality Inventory-2 (MMPI-2), 137, 162–163
MIRECCs (VA Mental Illness Research, Education, and Clinical Centers), 166–167
MMSE (Mini Mental-State Exam), 190
Model fidelity, 52

Modification, of EBPs, 27–32
Monitoring, 56, 70, 163
Monoamine oxidase inhibitors (MAOIs), 104
Motivation Assessment Scale (MAS), 137

Narcotics Anonymous, 181
NAs (nursing assistants), 195
National Coalition on Mental Health and Aging, 7
National Council on the Aging, 175
National Family Caregiver Support Program, 170
National Health Service of the United Kingdom, 222–223
National Institute of Mental Health, 6, 106
National Institute on Neurological Disorders and Stroke, 138
National Institutes of Mental Health Epidemiologic Catchment Area Study, 181
National Resource Center for Rural Elderly (NRCRE), 199, 201
Networking, 6–7
Neuroleptics, 113
Nevada Caregiver Support Center, 170
Nightingale, Florence, 179
NIH Consensus Statement on the Diagnosis of Dementia, 138
NMDA (N-Methyl-D-Asparate) receptor antagonists, 141
Nomothetic *versus* idiographic assessment, 162–163
Novak, Joseph D., 55
NRCRE (National Resource Center for Rural Elderly), 201
Nursing assistants (NAs), 195
Nursing home care. *See* Extended care

Obsessive compulsive disorder, 116
Olanzapine (Zyprexa), 139, 150–151
Older Adult and Family Center (Palo Alto), 170
Online resources, 5–6, 8*t. See also* Web sites
Opinion leaders, 39, 43

Opportunity costs, 23
Organizations, 18–22, 28
OTC (over-the-counter) drug abuse, 121
Outcome evaluation, 61–63, 62t, 78–79
Output costs, 25
Over-the-counter (OTC) drug abuse,
    121

PACE (Programs of All-Inclusive Care
    for the Elderly), 170–171
Panel on Cost-Effectiveness in Health
    and Medicine, 23, 24
Panic disorder, 115
PARC (Positive Aging Resource Center),
    6, 215–216
PARC TCE. See Positive Aging Resource
    Center, Targeted Capacity
    Expansion (PARC TCE) program
Partners in Caregiving (PIC), 193
Pascua Yaqui group, 69, 71, 74, 77
PATCH (Psychogeriatric Assessment and
    Treatment in City Housing), 173
Paykel Suicide Scale, 189
PDCA (Plan-Do-Check-Act) cycle,
    52–53
Peer counseling, 199–200
Peer review/editing process, 4
Phobias, 115–116
PIC (Partners in Caregiving), 193
Plan-Do-Check-Act (PDCA) cycle,
    52–53
Planning, 57–59, 70, 210
Political barriers to implementation, 29
Positive Aging Act (2002), 175
Positive Aging Resource Center (PARC),
    6, 215–216
Positive Aging Resource Center,
    Targeted Capacity Expansion
    (PARC TCE) program, 6, 68, 175
Posttraumatic Diagnostic Scale, 112
Posttraumatic stress disorder (PTSD),
    111–112, 116
Practice Guidelines from the International
    Society for Traumatic Stress Studies,
    116
Practitioners, culture of, 67, 73f, 82, 88
Presentations, as a community
    engagement technique, 75

President's New Freedom Commission
    on Mental Health, 168
Prevention of Suicide in Primary Care
    Elderly Collaborative Trial
    (PROSPECT), 168, 191
Primary care
    co-location of services and
        collaboration, 191–192
    effectiveness for mental health
        problems, 181–182
    integrated health care (See Integrated
        care)
    specialty mental health referral,
        188–191
    Web site, 203
Primary Care Research in Substance
    Abuse and Mental Health Services
    for the Elderly (PRISM-E), 172,
    175, 185
Principle fidelity, 52
PRISM-E (Primary Care Research in
    Substance Abuse and Mental Health
    Services for the Elderly), 172, 175,
    185
Problem solving, in quality
    management, 52–56
Process evaluation, 59–60t
Professional organizations and
    conferences, 6–7
Programs of All-Inclusive Care for the
    Elderly (PACE), 170–171
Prohaska, Jack, 80–82
Project A.W.A.R.E (Pennsylvania), 200
Promotions, as incentives, 49
Proposition 63 "Millionaire Tax"
    (California), 1
PROSPECT (Prevention of Suicide in
    Primary Care Elderly Collaborative
    Trial), 168, 191
PSA (psychosocial activities), 196
Psychoeducational groups, 187
Psychogeriatric Assessment and
    Treatment in City Housing
    (PATCH), 173
Psychogeriatric Rural Elderly Outreach
    Program (Virginia), 199
Psychosocial activities (PSA), 196
Psychotropic drugs, 139–142, 184

PsycInfo, 4, 5
PTSD (posttraumatic stress disorder), 111–112, 116
PubMed, 4

QALY (quality-adjusted life year), 24–25
QM (quality management). *See* Quality management (QM)
Quality-adjusted life year (QALY), 24–25
Quality control, 39
Quality indicators, 46–49, 47*t*
Quality management (QM)
  administrative strategy for, 38
  assessment of performance, 50–52
  evaluation strategies, 38, 56–63
  fishbone diagrams, 45*t*–46
  flowcharts, 44–45
  indicators and standards of quality, 46–49
  leadership, 37–38
  problem solving, 52–56
  as a system model, 38
  system support, 49–50
  teamwork, 37
  teamwork and, 38–44, 41*t*
Quetiapine (Seroquel), 139

Race/ethnicity, 9, 50, 146
Rapport building, 88, 90
Readiness assessment, 17–21, 60
Referral models, 165, 188–191
Registered nurse (RN), 192
Relapse, 153, 187
Relational ties, CG EBPs and, 71–72
Relaxation training, 114, 142
Religion, effect on behavioral health, 179
Reminyl (galantamine), 140
Research
  advisory committees, 33
  consultants, 7
  literature search, 4–8*t*
  locating toolkits, guidelines, or manuals, 5
  online information, 5–6
  professional organizations and conferences, 6–7

Resistance to change, 43
Rewards. *See* Incentives
Risk assessment, 27
Risperdal (risperidone), 139, 150–151
Rivastigmine (Exelon), 140
RN (registered nurse), 192
Rorshach test, 150
Rural Mental Health Work Group (NIMH), 198
Rural settings
  barriers to service delivery, 197–199
  definition of "rural," 197
  Health Improvement Program for the Elderly, 79–84
  integrated care systems, 185
  models of service delivery, 199–202

SAMHSA (Substance Abuse and Mental Health Services Administration), 5, 6, 70, 171, 174, 175, 220
Schizophrenia
  assessment, 147–150
  basic facts about, 146–148
  drug holidays, 153
  ineffective assessments, 150
  instruments for assessment, 149*t*
  medical treatments, 150–151
  psychosocial treatments, 151–152
  relapse/suicide prevention, 153
  selecting among treatments, 152–153
  self-help treatments (books and Web sites), 152
Screening, 121, 160–161, 186
Search engines, 4
Selection
  alternative use of EP or SIP, 13–14
  decision making in, 4*f*, 9–13
  identifying the target community, 3
  logic model for, 2*f*
  with no evidence for the target demographic group, 13
  researching, 3–8
Selective serotonin reuptake inhibitors (SSRIs), 104
Self-checking, for performance assessment, 51
Self-guided learning, 60
Self-help, 106, 152, 180–181

Self-managed work teams (SMWT), 194
Self-talk, 114
Seroquel (quetiapine), 139
Serotonin/norepinephrine reuptake
    inhibitors (SNRIs), 104
Service delivery
    assessment, 161–164 (*See also*
        Assessment)
·   collaborative care models for
        dementia, 169–170
    collaborative care models for
        depression, 167–168
    collaborative care models for severe
        mental illness, 168–169
    co-location models, 166–167 (*See also*
        Co-location)
    community-based outreach programs,
        166
    comparison studies, 172
    integrated care, 164–166 (*See also*
        Integrated care)
    prevention and outreach, 172–174
    Programs of All-Inclusive Care for the
        Elderly (PACE), 170–171
    screening, 121, 160–161, 186
    state-based programs for dual
        diagnosis, 171
Service-informed practice (SIP), 1, 13
Severe mental illness (SMI),
    collaborative care models for,
        168–169
Shewhart, Walter, 52
Short Michigan Alcohol Screening Test,
    189
Side effects, 107, 113, 150
SIP (service-informed practice), 1, 13
6-5-3 procedure, 46
Sleep deprivation, 119
SMI (severe mental illness),
    collaborative care models for,
        168–169
SMWT (self-managed work teams), 194
SNRIs (serotonin/norepinephrine
    reuptake inhibitors), 104
Social phobia, 116, 117
Social skills training, 151–152
Socioeconomic status, 74, 87

Somatic (behavioral health) factors, 90
Specialty mental health referral,
    188–191
Spokane Elderly Care Program, 199
SSRIs (selective serotonin reuptake
    inhibitors), 104
Stadick, Elizabeth, 76–77
Staff
    conventional staff management
        (CSM), 196
    culture of, 73t, 82, 88
    formal staff management (FSM), 196
    readiness for change, 19–20
    training, 186, 193, 195–197
    turnover in extended care settings,
        192–194
    web sites, 193, 194
    work setting culture and, 11
Standards, for quality improvement,
    46–49, 47t
Stanford Older Adult and Family Center,
    6
State-based programs for dual diagnosis,
    171
State programs for rural older adults,
    171, 200–202
State/Trait Anxiety Scale, 83t, 84t
Stereotypes, 69, 93
Stigmatization, 90, 184, 191, 192, 197
Structured Clinical Interview for DSM–IV,
    111, 162
Substance Abuse and Mental Health
    Services Administration
    (SAMHSA), 5, 6, 70, 171, 174, 220
Substance use disorders
    Alcoholics Anonymous (AA) and,
        180, 191
    anxiety disorders and, 110, 113, 116
    assessment of, 120–121
    basic facts about, 118–120
    depression and, 100
    interventions for, 121–123
Suicide, 100, 148, 153, 181, 189
Supervision, 20, 21, 54, 55t
Surviving Schizophrenia: A Manual for
    Families, Consumers, and Providers,
    152

Sustainability
  defining, 211–213
  determining effectiveness, 209–210
  factors, 214t, 216t
  implementation and, 215–217
  the Kajsiab House program, 217–221
  planning for, 210–211
  predicting, 211–213, 222
  tips for creation of, 221–223
  Web sites, 222
System-control model. *See* Quality
    management (QM)
System support, 49–50

Tacrine (Cognex), 140
Targeted Capacity Expansion (TCE)
    grant program, 6, 68, 175
Target population(s), identifying, 3, 13,
    70
TAT (Thematic Apperception Test), 150
TCAs (tricyclic antidepressants), 104,
    108
TCE (Targeted Capacity Expansion)
    grant program, 6, 68, 175
Teams, 37, 38–44, 41t, 51
Thematic Apperception Test (TAT), 150
Theoretical/principle-based barriers to
    implementation, 28–29
Thioridazine, 150
Tiempo de Oro (Phoenix)
  applying the CG EBP model, 75–79
  between-group differences and, 68, 69
  language and communication, 71, 74
  relational ties, 71–72
  values and belief systems, 72
  within-group differences and, 69
Toolkits, 5
Tools, quality management (QM), 54–56
Training
  costs of, 26
  culture of work setting and staff and,
    11
  for extended care staff, 193, 195–197
  for integrated care staff, 186
  level needed, 29–30
  organizational climate and, 21

of primary care professionals by
    behavioral health professionals, 165
  resource readiness and, 20
Trauma Symptom Inventory, 112
Trazadone, 104
Tricyclic antidepressants (TCAs), 104,
    108
Trochim, William, 55
Turnover, 192–194
Twelve-step programs, 180, 191

United States Air Force, 185
University of Arizona Center on Aging,
    70

VA community-based outpatient clinics,
    185
Values, 20, 21, 72, 87, 217
VA Mental Illness Research, Education,
    and Clinical Centers (MIRECCs),
    166–167
Vang, Doua, 218–221
Vascular dementia, 135, 140
Veterans Affairs (VA), 166–167, 185
VISNs (Veterans Integrated Service
    Networks), 167

WebMD Depression Health Center, 106
Web sites
  Alzheimer's disease, 145
  Axon Idea Processor, 55–56
  concept mapping, 55
  data collection system, 70, 83
  dementia, 146
  depression, 106
  evaluation consultants, 57
  faith-based programs, 202–203
  FDA, 140
  LEAP, 195
  literature searches, 4–8t
  Network for the Improvement of
    Addiction Treatment, 222
  primary care, 203
  SAMHSA, 175
  schizophrenia, 152
  staff turnover, 193, 194
  state of Oregon, 223

Web sites (*cont.*)
  sustainability, 222, 223
  VA Mental Illness Research,
    Education, and Clinical Centers
    (MIRECCs), 167
  Wellspring Model, 194
Wellspring Model, 194–195
Wernicke's encephalopathy, 119

Within-group heterogeneity, 69, 88
Workshops, as a community
    engagement technique, 75–76, 79

Yoga, 114

Ziprasidone (Geodon), 139
Zyprexa (olanzapine), 139